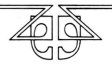
Atlas of the Newborn

Neil O'Doherty

MD, FRCP, DCH
The Children's Hospital
Temple Street, Dublin

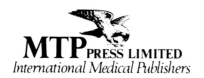
MTP PRESS LIMITED
International Medical Publishers

To Angela

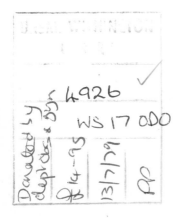

Published by
MTP Press Limited
Falcon House, Lancaster, England

ISBN-0-85200-236–X

Printed in Great Britain by Waterlow (Dunstable) Ltd.

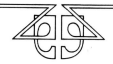

Atlas of the Newborn

Contents

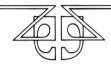

Foreword

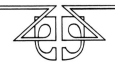

An Atlas of the Newborn is long overdue. Anyone with experience in the nursery realizes that observation is the essential approach to evaluation of the newborn. What is it one observes? Obviously it is size and shape, it is activity and, most importantly perhaps, skin and its appendages. Gestational age can be deduced from developmental stages of the skin; state of oxygenation from skin colour; and many major and minor malformations are associated with skin tags, dimples, extra digits or other readily observable abnormalities. A surprising deficiency in the medical literature (now overcome) has been a collection of colour photographs of the obvious signs that could be useful to the student of the newborn.

A trip to any of our medical libraries would make it apparent that there is a burgeoning literature relevant to the normal and abnormal newborn infant. This literature is expressed first in the form of publications in journals, then proceedings of symposia which try to establish the state of the art, and, as in all fields, finally compilations of information in the form of textbooks. Some of these textbooks started as single-authored but quickly became multi-authored as the amount of information that seemed important to convey exceeded the capacity of any individual to convey with great authority. Despite the proliferation of words, good colour photographs are rare.

One wonders why a colour atlas of the normal and abnormal newborn has been so long in coming. Perhaps it awaited a careful observer with a good camera and a willing publisher. At any rate, it is now our good fortune that Dr. Neil O'Doherty has undertaken this assignment. He has organized his approach under the following headings: "The Normal Infant and his Trivial Complaints", "Low-Birth-Weight Babies", "Trauma", "Infection", "Congenital Abnormality", and "Skin Defects". Dr. O'Doherty has collected a superb group of coloured photographs, and added a commentary which precedes the collection of photos.

The special qualities of this particular book are the numbers of colour photographs which illustrate as words never can the findings of interest. An atlas such as this shares with all atlases the features of being a road map which allows one to establish a starting point. Other sources can then be approached for further discussion on pathogenesis and management. Unlike most publications, this work has little chance of becoming substantially out of date.

The observations presented here are timeless and are reproduced in most every active nursery every year. It seems improbable that the kinds of malformations, injuries, or lesions depicted will change significantly in the decades or even centuries to come.

Dr. O'Doherty has made a major contribution for his contemporaries; it is almost certain that future generations of neonatologists and perinatologists will continue to refer to this careful collection of observations.

Mary Ellen Avery, M.D.

THOMAS MORGAN ROTCH PROFESSOR OF PEDIATRICS
HARVARD MEDICAL SCHOOL
PHYSICIAN-IN-CHIEF
CHILDREN'S HOSPITAL MEDICAL CENTER, BOSTON, MASSACHUSETTS

Preface

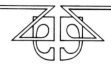

Today more than four-fifths of all deliveries in the British Isles take place in hospital, where routine paediatric surveillance and care are available for all babies. Yet it is scarcely a generation since it began to be accepted that there should be a paediatric presence at the birth or in the early days of every baby and in these few years the outlook for the newborn child has been transformed.

The dramatic initial impact came through the introduction of antibiotics, exchange transfusion, and the possibility of safe major surgery; more recently there has been a spreading appreciation of the benefits of universal screening to detect conditions ranging from hip instability to phenylketonuria.

Such advances, important as they are, help only a minority of babies, and they must therefore be viewed in perspective. For the great majority of babies the most pressing immediate daily need is for improvements in the quality of the routine care given by the clinical services in the neonatal period. It is in these days and weeks that the human child is at highest risk, and he or she undergoes what are likely to be the most important routine examinations of a whole lifetime. No other set examination reveals so much that requires explanation or action. At no stage in life are the rewards higher for the preventive clinical approach. A thorough neonatal examination as a matter of routine should be one of the child's inalienable rights.

There is a basic problem at the outset. Most newborn babies are healthy, and only a relatively small number of doctors come to acquire a significant neonatal commitment in the ordinary way. In this sphere, medical school curricula are unable to do more than sketch out the fundamentals of care in the course of teaching undergraduates the sound principles of practical management.

A doctor will enjoy neonatal work only if he develops an interest in it and acquires an initial confidence in his ability to cope with situations as they arise. This interest comes from the recognition of each baby's individuality and of the fact that he is the sum of his inheritance and life-experience to date. Confidence is based on his ability to distinguish trivial complaints from the subtle early signs of disaster and to recognise pointers to imminent danger.

It is with the aim of promoting knowledge and confidence in recognising the various visual aspects of the newborn that this Atlas is published.

This book has been prepared with the cooperation of the Departments of Paediatrics and Medical Photography at the West Middlesex Hospital and Guy's Hospital, London. Dr. Stephen Lamb kindly advised on the textual content of section four (Infection) and permitted the use of illustrations 3 and 4 in this section. Dr. Janet Hardy and the Johns Hopkins Collaborative Perinatal Study kindly permitted the use of illustration 55 in section five (Congenital Abnormality). Diagrams and drawings by Susan Robinson, Department of Medical Illustration, West Middlesex Hospital, London.

Section one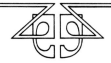

The normal infant and his trivial complaints

Introduction

The first and most important part of the initial routine examination of the newborn is a thorough and systematic inspection of the baby's external appearance. This can reveal wide individual variations and yet remain within the normal range. A sound knowledge of the range of normal is the foundation on which the doctor can manage the average newborn baby with safety, confidence and enjoyment. Attention is directed to the postural and compressional effects of prenatal and intrapartum influences, to the skin, the mouth, sexual characteristics, and the navel together with the cord.

1-4

When the baby is in a good state of arousal the normal posture is one of dominant flexion (1) with the limbs supported off the examining surface. If the baby is barely awake (2) the limbs normally rest on the surface. If this occurs when the baby is in a higher state of arousal, it is a non-specific sign of malaise (3: infant of diabetic mother; 4: after emergency Caesarean section) usually caused by hypotonia or weakness. In its most florid form it is called the (pithed) 'frog posture'.

5-7

Limb posture is normally affected temporarily when the head lies in the lateral position (5, 6); the mental limbs extend and the occipital limbs flex (it is called the asymmetrical tonic neck response, or the 'fencer' posture). Occasionally, as a normal variation, the opposite can occur – mental limbs flex and occipital limbs extend (7). If asymmetrical tonic neck postures are strongly imposed some neurological disorder may exist.

8-12

Abnormal presentations show tell-tale postural effects in the neck hyperextension of face or brow (8) and in the way the lower limbs are held after flexed or extended breech (9, 10). In any breech birth, the head is not moulded and the vertex is flattened with occipital overhang (11). This is in contrast with average normal axial moulding (12) which is most obvious in first pregnancies following prolonged engagement of the head.

13-15

The feet can be moulded into postural talipes (13) which is fully mobile (14) and the 'position of ease' demonstrated soon after birth (15).

16-20

Ear-to-shoulder compression is common. The mother may notice that the mandible is pushed up on the compressed side (16), but this straightens within weeks or at the most a few months. The side of the neck is excavated and the lower pinna sticks out if it has been caught on the point of the shoulder (17). The nose may be squashed out of shape (18) and even the vault may be a little crooked (19). These all straighten in due course. The compressed sternomastoid muscle, however, may develop a 'tumour' from ischaemic necrosis; this will not be seen in the nursery as it does not appear until the end of the second week (20); the condition must be watched because torticollis may develop. In extreme cases there may be congenital facial palsy, which may persist.

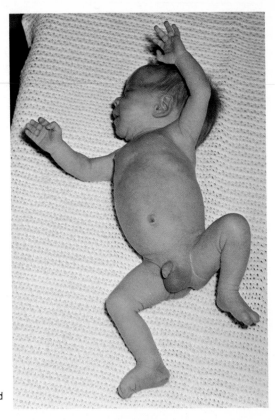

1. Posture of the normal aroused infant

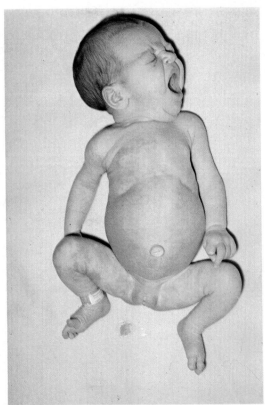

2. Posture of the normal infant when barely awake

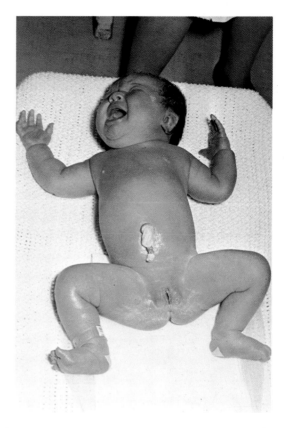

3. Infant of a diabetic mother

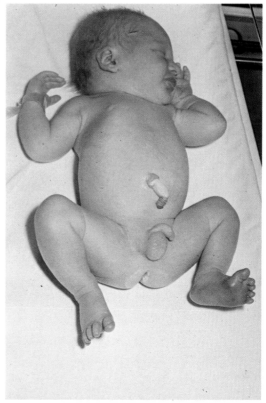

4. Infant after emergency Cæsarean section

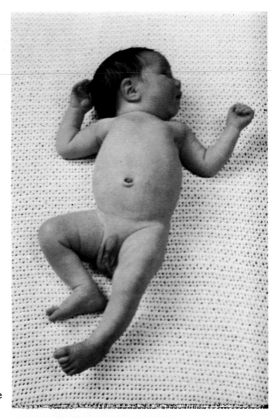

5. Asymmetrical tonic neck response
with the head turned to the left

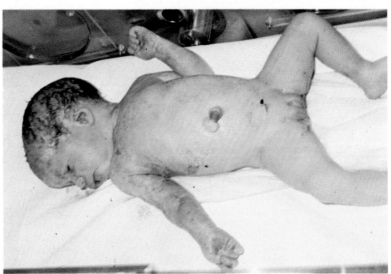

6. Asymmetrical tonic neck response
with the head turned to the right

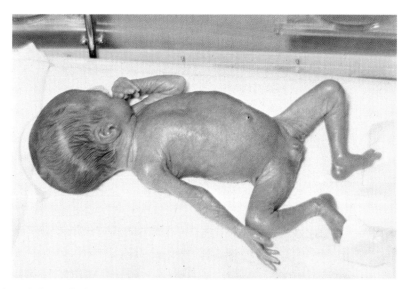

7. Normal variation of the asymmetrical tonic neck response

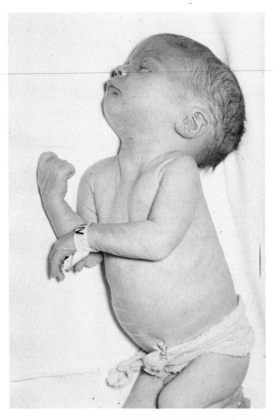

8. Hyperextension of the neck after brow presentation

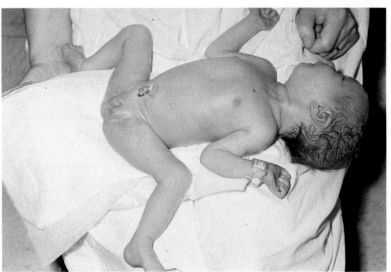

9. Limb position following breech presentation with flexed lower limbs

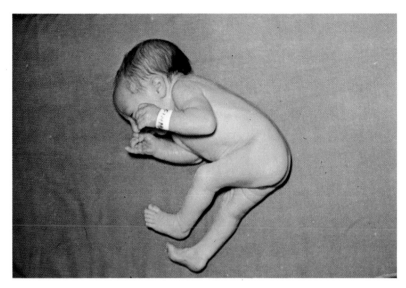

10. Limb position following breech presentation with extended lower limbs

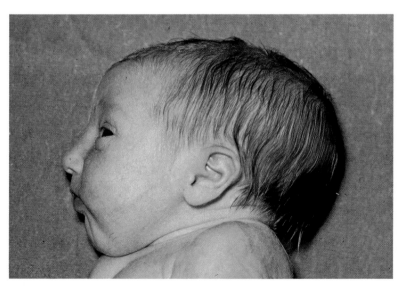

11. Flattened vertex and occipital overhang following breech presentation

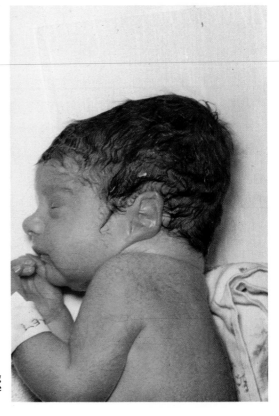

12. Average normal axial moulding
following prolonged engagement of the
head

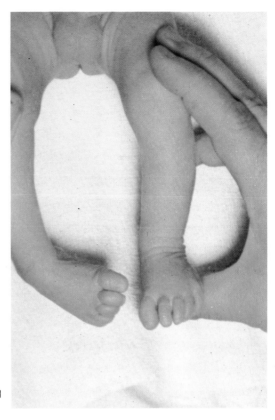

13. Moulding of the feet into postural talipes

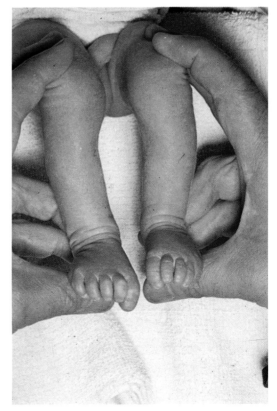

14. Full mobility of postural talipes

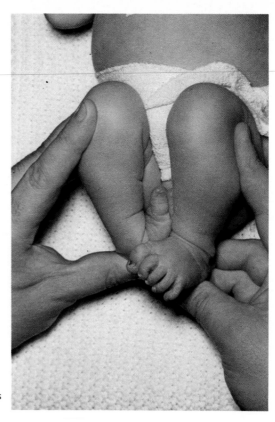

15. Position of ease in postural talipes demonstrated soon after birth

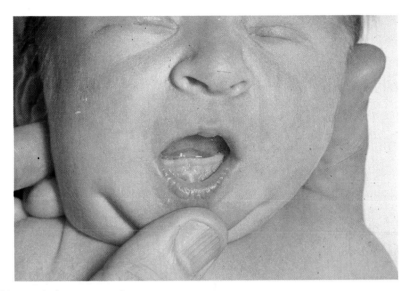

16. Mandible pushed up on the compressed side following ear-to-shoulder compression

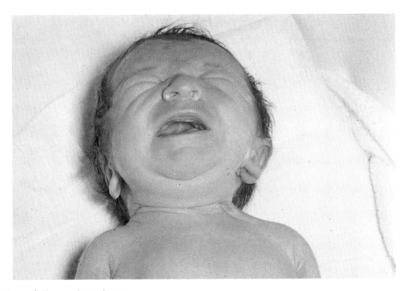

17. Excavation of the neck and protruding lower pinna following ear-to-shoulder compression

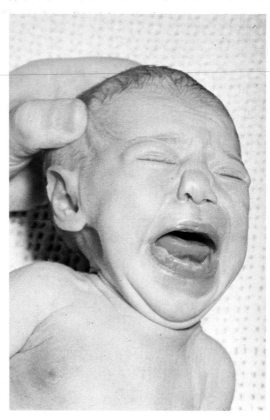

18. Squashing of the nose in ear-to-shoulder compression

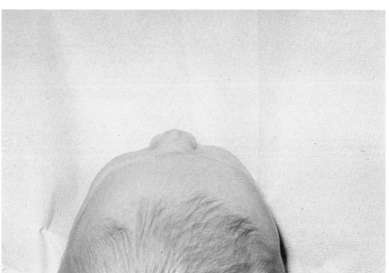

19. Crooked vault following intra-uterine compression

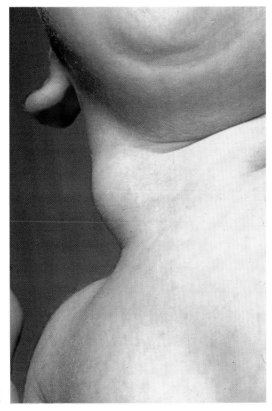

20. "Tumour" from ischaemic necrosis
of the compressed Sternomastoid muscle

This is a very striking feature, its condition and appearance can change remarkably from day to day and at first even from hour to hour. It is essential to be able to recognise this secular variation if the normal range is to be fully understood; for it is upon such understanding that early diagnosis of abnormality is based, and without this understanding many false alarms will be raised.

21, 22, 29   *Vernix caseosa*

At birth there is a cheesy white deposit, *vernix caseosa*, which may be liberally caked all over (21) or concentrated in folds like the groins (22) or behind the ears (29). Vernix normally dries out and flakes off within a few hours. No attempt need therefore be made to remove it. The presence of vernix indicates that the baby is not many hours old and that gestation was at, or close to, term. Its white colour can alter in conditions of fetal pathology to a golden-yellow in postmaturity or erythroblastosis, or it may be stained by meconium or bile passed because of fetal distress in utero.

22-32   Peripheral cyanosis

Erythema neonatorum

Harlequin colour change

The palms and soles (22, 28, 29) and the circumoral area (23) are often blue at birth and this peripheral cyanosis is acceptable as normal during the first 48 hours of life if the general condition is satisfactory and there is no evidence of central cyanosis, i.e. warm parts like the tongue will be pink. This 'normal' cyanosis has a lavender hue which can deepen to damson if the baby is unwell, for instance after the anoxic experience of a difficult delivery (24). Gentle stroking induces a rapid vasomotor reaction resulting in sudden dispersal of peripheral cyanosis (25, 26). In babies more than a couple of days old the appearance of peripheral cyanosis is a non-specific sign of illness which may be due to a number of causes including infection or heart-failure (27). The baby's general condition is poor and cyanosis developing at this stage has a flatter, slaty colour which may be accentuated by accompanying pallor. Soon after birth, the scrotal skin is cherry-coloured in contrast with the pinkness of more central skin areas (28). When the baby is several hours old, a brilliant red flush often develops all over the body. This is *erythema neonatorum* (29) or the 'boiled lobster' effect whose angry look must not be mistaken for inflammation – it fades within 24 hours. At some time during the first few days of life a vivid line of demarcation may appear down the midline (30) or in rare instances it may be transverse. This is the harlequin colour change, a striking but innocuous vasomotor phenomenon. A marked colour difference at birth between uniovular twins (31) may be due to homotransfusion prior to cord clamping, through vascular connections within the placenta (32: the arterial territories communicate at both poles) or between the two cords.

33-37		Some characteristics of the term baby's skin may be more common and more florid in the low-birth-weight baby. They include fine lanugo hair (33) on the body at birth or skin peeling after a few days (34). Meconium staining (35) results from fetal distress; the routine treatment is a stomach washout to remove any meconium that may have been swallowed. After the skin has been cleaned there may be residual evidence of fetal distress from a stained cord (36) or meconium ingrained around the nailbeds (37).
38, 39	Jaundice	Mild jaundice commonly occurs in term babies; it is related to a physiological bilirubin peak at about four days and its onset is rare before the second or after the seventh day. It usually disappears well before the child is two weeks old. This jaundice, with a good haemoglobin level, is orange in colour (38), unlike the jaundice associated with anaemia which is lemon in colour (39).
40, 41	*Erythema toxicum*	From about the second day skin lesions of the histamine-weal variety, like nettlerash (40, 41), are commonly observed. These are little papules or vesicles surrounded by a mild erythema (*erythema toxicum*) or 'flea-bite dermatitis'. In spite of their inflamed appearance the baby is well. In typical cases the lesions come and go in various sites on the trunk and the limbs before they disappear by the end of the first week. They are unusual in the first 24 hours and are rarely congenital; they are not seen in pre- or post-term babies. The lesions usually spare the baby's face and this fact has led to the postulate that a cause of the condition is friction between skin and baby-clothes; this is strengthened by the fact that such lesions are not usually observed in a term baby nursed naked in an incubator. The fluid from a vesicle is rich in eosinophil cells, while the eosinophil level in the peripheral blood is normal.
42, 43	*Milia* Sudamina	On the face, especially in the muzzle area, there is usually a very fine raised eruption in the first few days. The small lesions, looking like grains of powder, are due to the accumulation of secretions in sebaceous glands and are called *milia* from a fancied resemblance to millet seeds (42: *milia*, a few show cystic dilatation). A little later, in the second week, blockage of sweat gland ducts may produce superficial vesicles of about pinhead size (43) called sudamina. The newborn baby does not sweat efficiently, and the rash is commonest in hot weather.

44-47

Stork marks

Port wine stain

Naevus flammeus

Naevi caused by capillary dilatation are common on the upper lids and across the glabella (44), down the nose, on the upper lip (45) and at the nape of the neck (46), where they have been given the fanciful name of 'stork marks'. The lesions fade gradually and have usually gone by the end of the second year. Those on the nape of the neck, however, are more liable to persist. Denser capillary naevi (port wine stains, *naevus flammeus*) (47) are less likely to fade but are usually innocuous. In certain locations, or distributions, they may, however, indicate underlying trouble, for example Sturge-Weber disease when the first or second division of the trigeminal nerve is involved.

48-54

Mongolian blue spot

A naevus caused by slaty-blue pigment deposited in the lower lumbar region is common in Negro or Asiatic children; it is called the Mongolian blue spot (48) – but has nothing to do with Down's syndrome of mongolism. If it measures much more than the usual few cms. across its distribution it is sometimes called 'bathing trunk' (49). Like the stork mark, it fades away gradually. Two comments are necessary. Firstly, where the pattern is 'universal' (50), it is possible for an uninitiated junior doctor keenly aware of the 'battered baby syndrome' to mistake it for extensive bruising. Secondly, in a fair-skinned baby (51) the pattern may point to racial admixture. In such cases one should inspect the genital skin which is darker in all races, and strikingly so in the coloured male (52) and female (53). One notices the in-between pigmentation typical of admixture (54) although this observation in itself would not bear medico-legal scrutiny.

55-63

Various tags (55, 56, 57, 58, 62), pits and dimples (59, 60, 61) are often present and usually are trivial. Careful checks, however, must always be carried out, because of the possibility of associated serious malformation, especially if the lesion is in a 'danger' area such as the lower lumbar region. Small tags with a very narrow peduncle can be tied off with black silk. They shrivel up and drop off after a few days. An exception is the vulval tag (63) which should be left alone because it soon vanishes spontaneously.

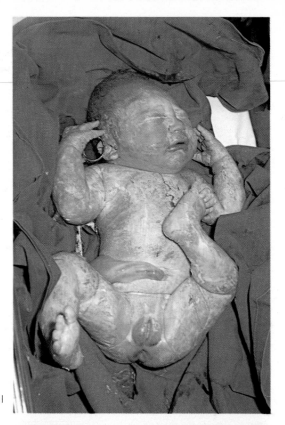

21. *Vernix caseosa* liberally caked all over the fetus

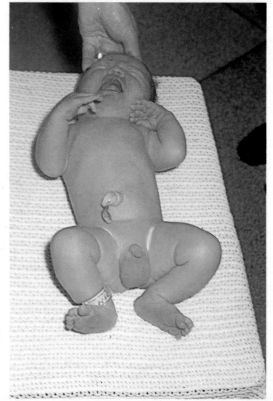

22. Residual *vernix caseosa* in the folds of the groin. The palms and soles show the lavender blue cyanosis which is normal during the first 48 hours

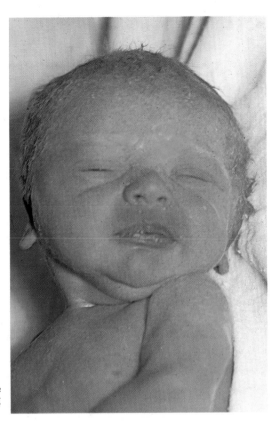

23. Lavender blue cyanosis of the
circumoral area which is normal during
the first 48 hours

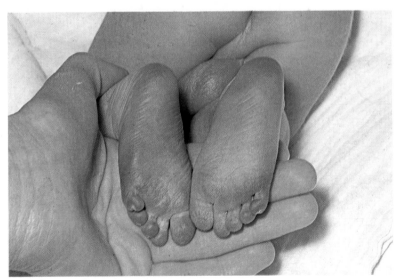

24. Deeper damson-coloured cyanosis
of the soles after anoxic experience of a
difficult delivery

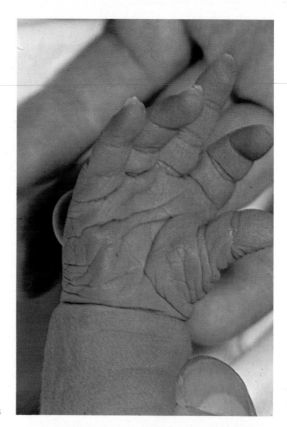

25. Palm showing peripheral cyanosis

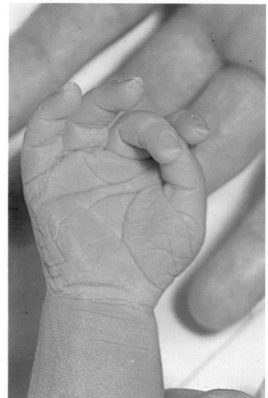

26. The same palm as in plate 25 after
sudden dispersal of peripheral cyanosis
induced by gentle stroking

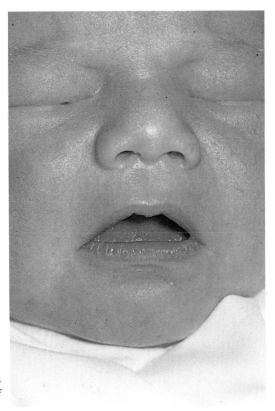

27. Peripheral cyanosis appearing after the first 48 hours as a non-specific sign of illness

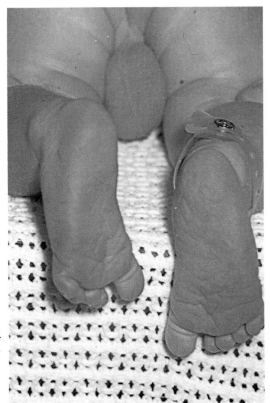

28. Cherry-coloured scrotal skin soon after birth contrasts with the pinkness of more central skin areas. The soles show evidence of peripheral cyanosis

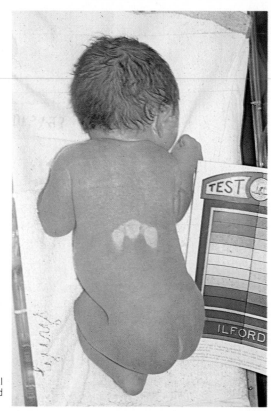

29. *Erythema neonatorum* and normal
lavender blue cyanosis of the palms and
soles

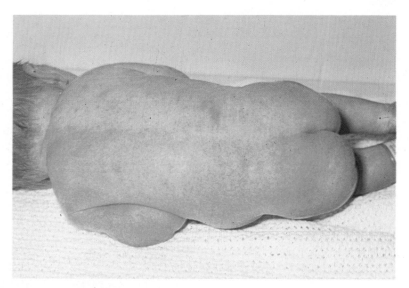

30. A vivid line of demarcation down
the midline: 'harlequin' colour change

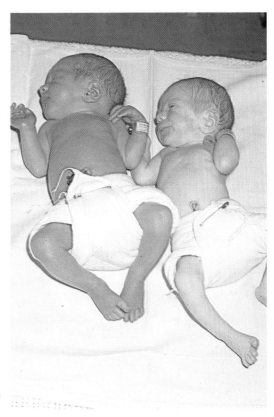

31. Marked colour difference at birth between uniovular twins

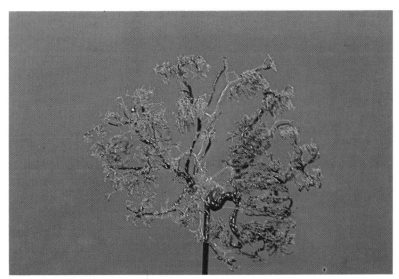

32. Vascular connections within the placenta showing arterial territories communicating at both poles

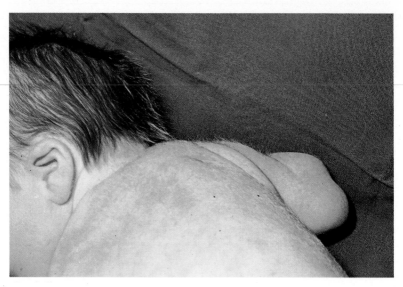

33. Fine lanugo hair at birth

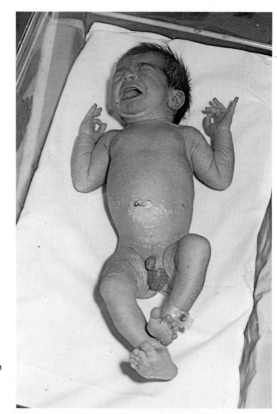

34. Peeling skin a few days after birth

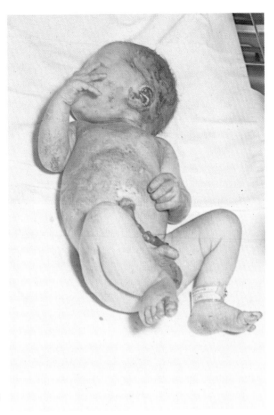

35. Meconium staining of the skin following fetal distress

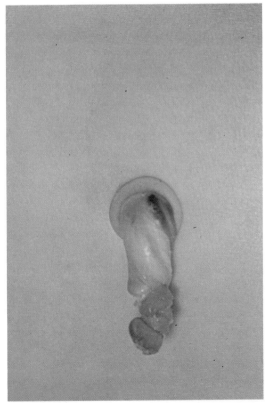

36. Meconium staining of the cord following fetal distress

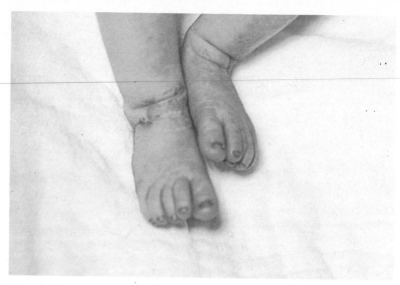

37. Meconium ingrained around the
nailbeds following fetal distress

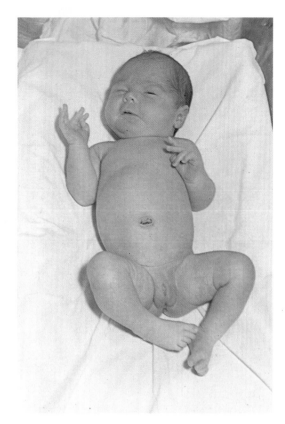

38. Physiological jaundice

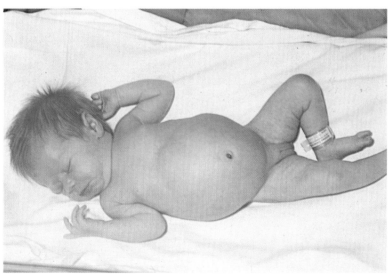

39. Jaundice associated with anaemia

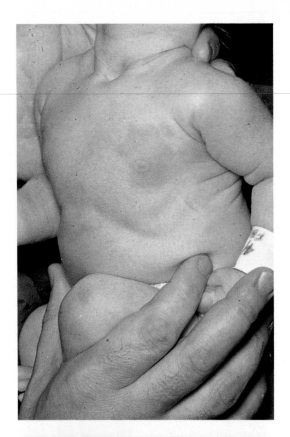

40. *Erythema toxicum*

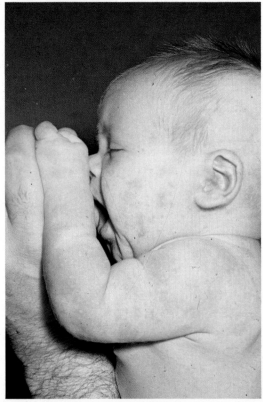

41. *Erythema toxicum*

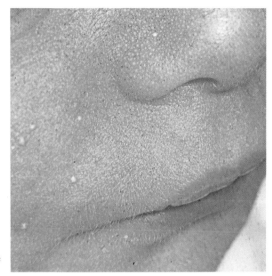

42. Milia: some of the larger lesions are cystic

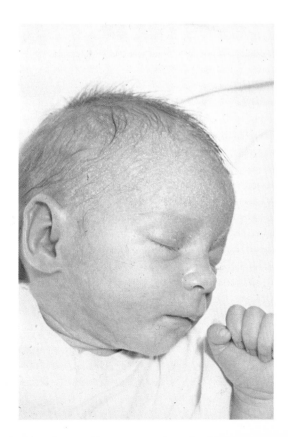

43. Sudamina

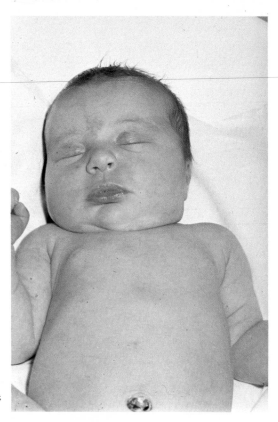

44. 'Stork marks' on the upper lids and the glabella

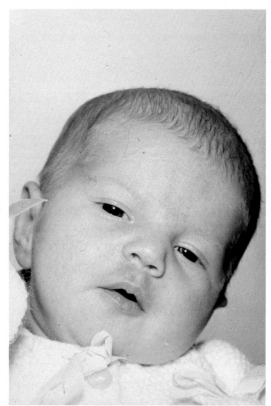

45. 'Stork marks' on the upper lip

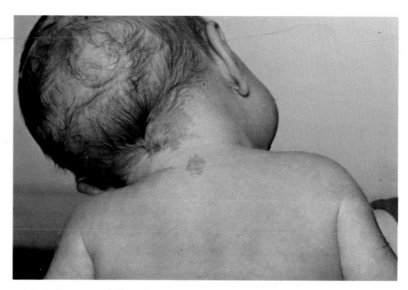

46. 'Stork marks' at the nape of the
neck

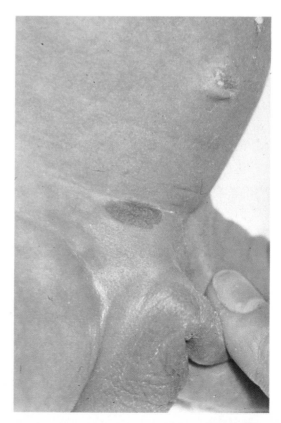

47. Port wine stain or naevus flammeus

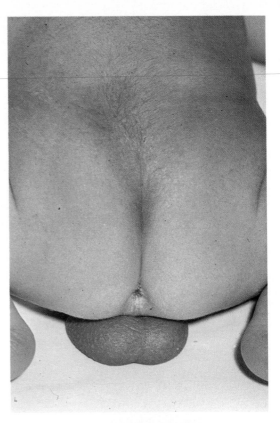

48. Mongolian blue spot

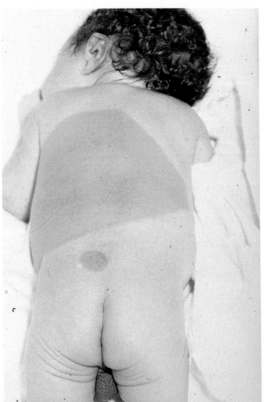

49. Larger   Mongolian   blue   spot:
'bathing trunk' distribution

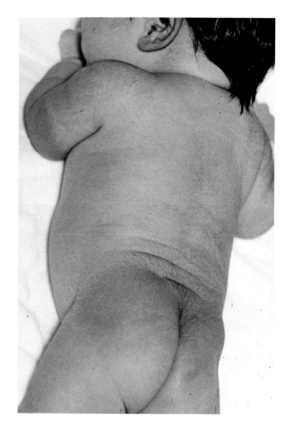

50. 'Universal' Mongolian blue spot

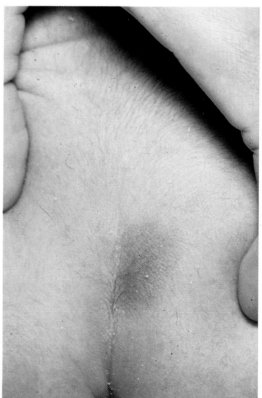

51. Mongolian blue spot in a fair-skinned baby

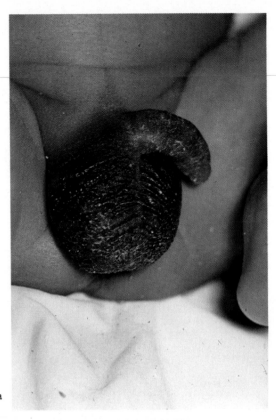

52. Strikingly darker genital skin of a
coloured male

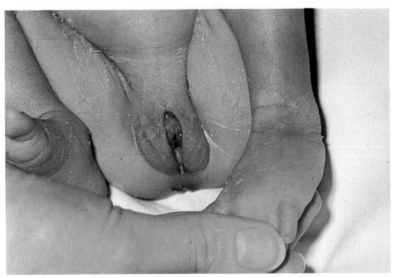

53. Strikingly darker genital skin of a
coloured female

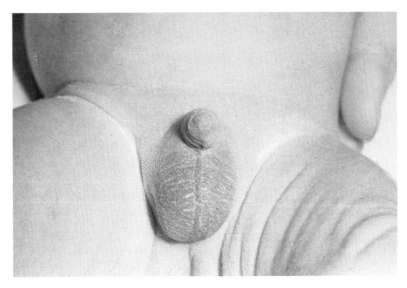

54. In-between pigmentation of the
genital skin typical of racial admixture

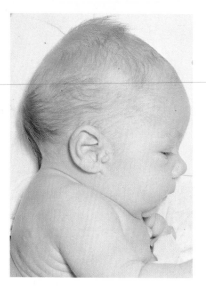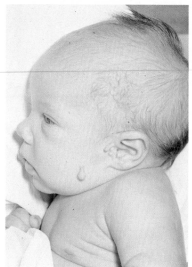

55. Facial tags

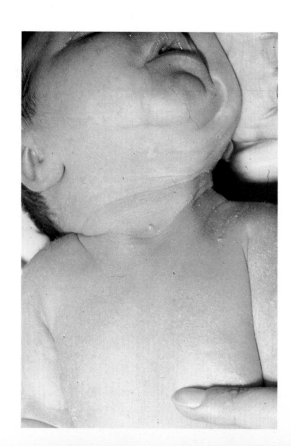

56. Tags on the neck

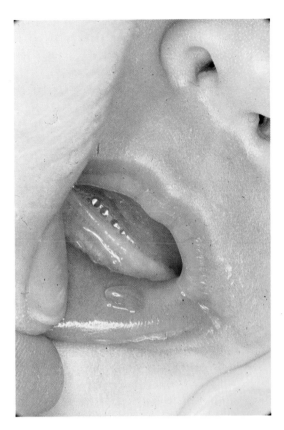

57. Tag on the inside of the lip

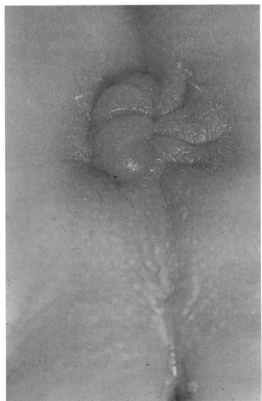

58. Perianal tag

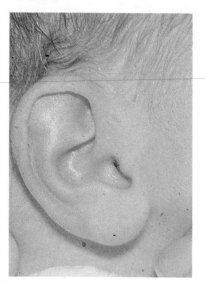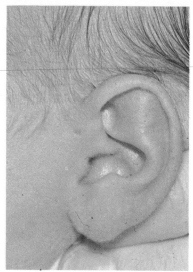

59. Preauricular pits

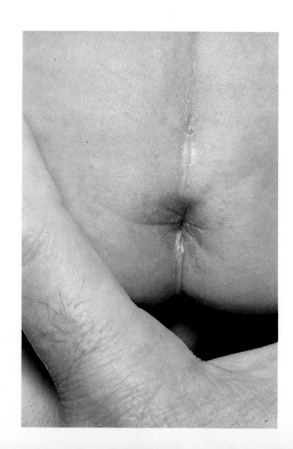

60. Deep sacrococcygeal pit

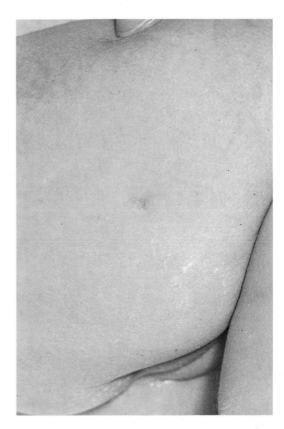

61. Dimple

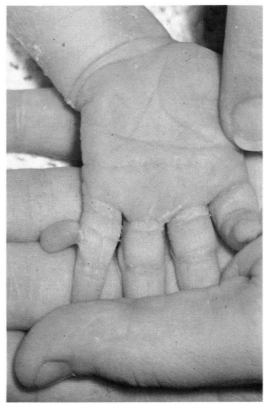

62. Rudimentary supernumerary digit

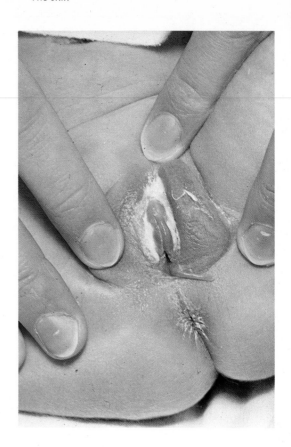

63. Vulval tag

64-66 Sucking callouses

From birth the lips show a demarcation line where the mucous membrane meets the skin portion (64). A few days later the surface is thrown up into folds or cushions called sucking 'callouses' (65). The word is a misnomer since these are not callosities due to pressure or friction. They have been seen at their most florid in a baby who had never sucked because of congenital heart disease (66). To suck efficiently, the newborn baby must form a complete seal with his lips around the nipple or teat. The 'callouses' resemble in appearance the lateral aspect of an index finger when the interphalangeal joints are flexed. As the 'callouses' are shed, new ones may crop for a few weeks.

67-70 Epithelial pearls

Epstein's pearls

Epithelial pearls are areas where the cells are condensed in whorls or small cysts. These are most often seen in the mouth: the commonest, called Epstein's pearls, consist of a small cluster at the junction of the soft and hard palate in the midline (67). They should be left alone as they soon fade away and efforts to rub them off with gauze can result in pterygoid ulcers as the delicate mucosa is rubbed over the underlying bone. Other pearls may be seen on the alveolar margin (68), on the areola (69), or on the foreskin (70).

71-73 Natal teeth

Epulis

Natal teeth may be present (71) commonly in the central incisor region, and there is a familial pattern of occurrence. They are usually only immature caps of enamel and dentine with poor root formation. It is best to remove them because they would soon exfoliate spontaneously and might be aspirated. They are nearly all from the normal deciduous complement and extraction will not deplete the permanent dentition. Sometimes an eruption cyst is observed on the gum at birth and the neonatal tooth appears shortly afterwards (72). A congenital epulis (73) occurs in the incisor region of the maxillary alveolar mucosa, usually in female babies. This is a form of embryonal hamartoma. The larger ones may have to be excised but the smaller resolve spontaneously.

74-76 *Ranula*

A superficial swelling known as a mucous cyst may appear in the anterior part of the floor of the mouth (74); some deeper cysts (75) occur in relation to the submandibular or sublingual ducts. Either may be called a *ranula* if the distended mucosa looks like the belly of a frog. The larger ones may need to be uncapped surgically but the smaller ones disappear either spontaneously or aided by needle puncture. They may be bilateral (76).

77

The lingual frenulum may be thick and the tongue tip dimpled (77). True tongue-tie, however, is a great rarity, hardly ever diagnosed in the newborn period; if such a frenulum is divided the tongue still rides close to the floor of the mouth.

78

The labial frenum similarly may be thickened and continuous with the median palatal raphe through an alveolar notch (78). Usually this is of no consequence. If, however, there is a diastema between the central incisors as the canines begin to erupt – between the ages of 9 and 11 years – the thickened frenum should be excised together with extension through the gap into the median raphe.

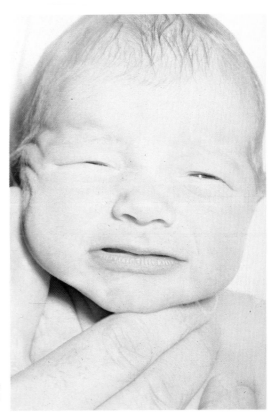

64. Demarcation line on the lips where the mucous membrane meets the skin portion

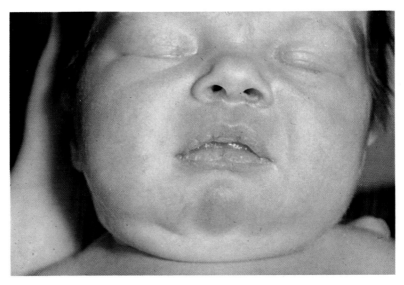

65. Sucking 'callouses'

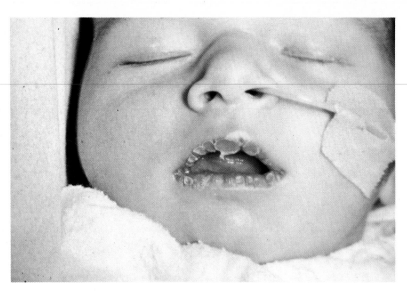

66. Sucking 'callouses' in a baby who
had never sucked

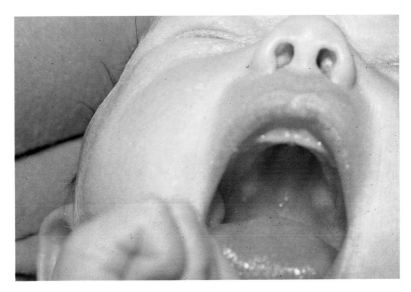

67. Epstein's pearls

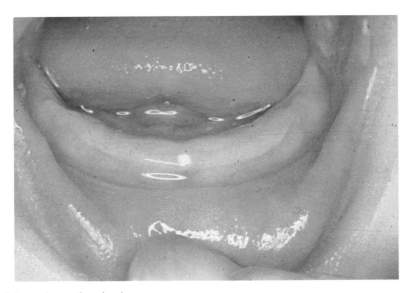

68. Epithelial pearl on the alveolar
margin

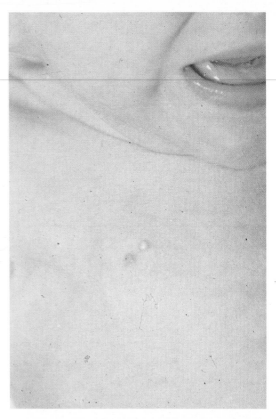

69. Pearl on the areola

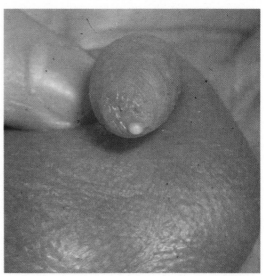

70. Pearl on the foreskin

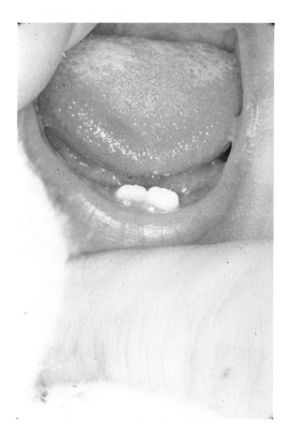

71. Natal teeth

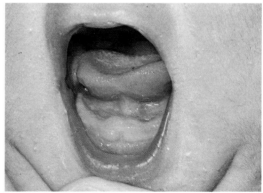

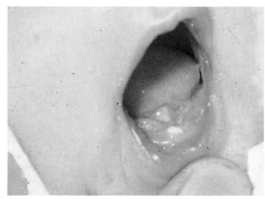

72. Dental eruption cysts on the gum at birth and the neonatal tooth which appeared shortly afterwards

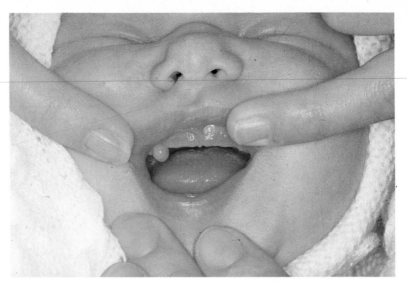

73. Congenital epulis

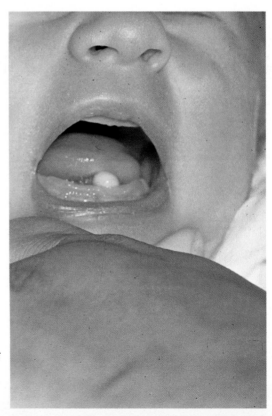

74. Mucous cyst in the anterior part of
the floor of the mouth

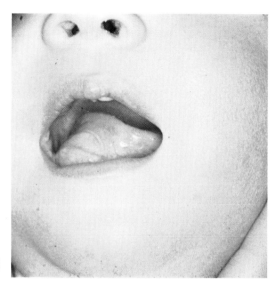

75. Deeper mucous cyst (*ranula*) associated with a sublingual duct

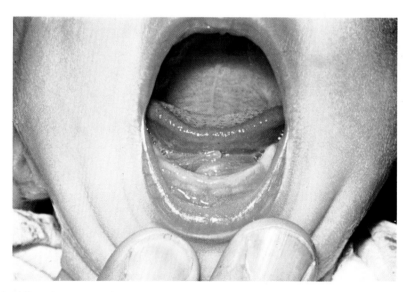

76. Bilateral sublingual mucous cysts

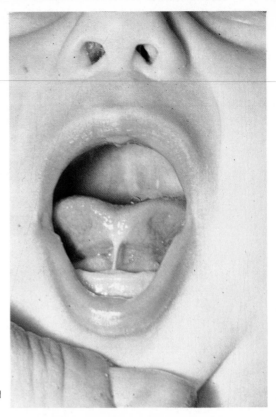

77. Thick lingual frenulum and dimpled
tongue tip

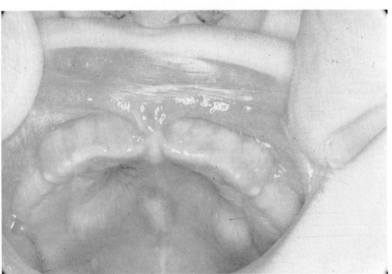

78. Labial frenum thickened and continuous with the median palatal raphe

The genitalia of the newborn female baby gape slightly, partially uncovering the labia minora and perhaps the clitoris (79). Mucoid vaginal secretion is common (80). The clitoris is large and in pre-term babies so large that the inexperienced practitioner may suspect intersex. In the newborn male, the relatively large size of the phallus makes the baby appear 'well endowed'.

Transplacental hormonal effects occur. Withdrawal bleeding from the vagina (81) may start on the third or fourth day and go on for two or three days. Both sexes are equally liable to breast enlargement (82). After two or three days the hypertrophied breasts may become engorged and a form of lactation occurs – 'witch's milk' (83) – which can be expressed. The swelling begins to subside in the second week and has usually gone by the third or fourth week, but it is more persistent in girls and may remain for several months (84: age 6 months). While it is present, the stagnant milk predisposes to infection as in mothers who stop nursing, and these infants are liable to mastitis or abscess formation. Supernumerary nipples (85) are commonly seen below and slightly medial to the breasts. They usually have no glandular tissue (86: in a mother near term). They may be multiple (87).

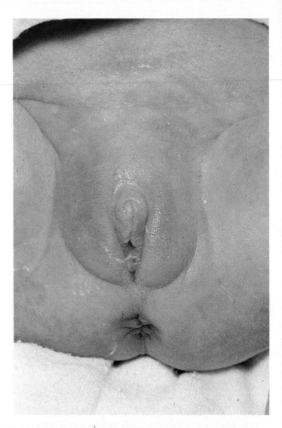

79. Genitalia of the newborn female

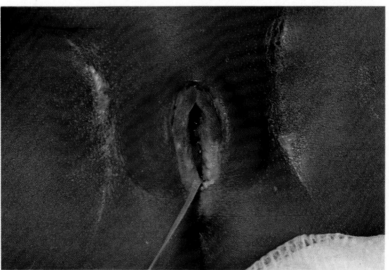

80. Mucoid vaginal secretion

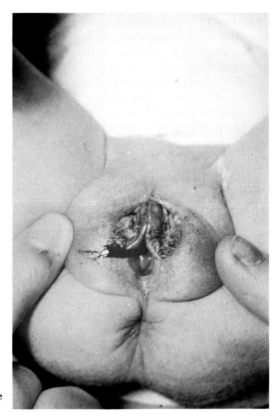

81. Withdrawal bleeding from the vagina

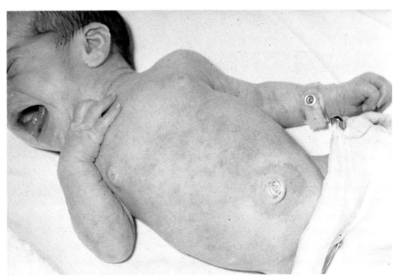

82. Breast enlargement

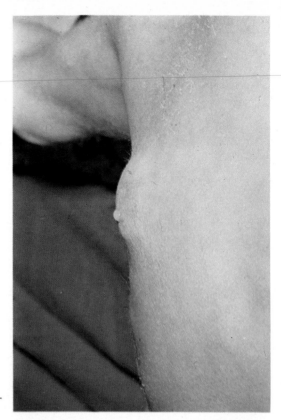

83. 'Witch's milk' from hypertrophied breast tissue

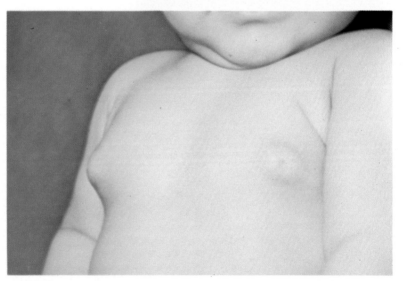

84. A six month old baby girl with
persistent swelling of the breasts

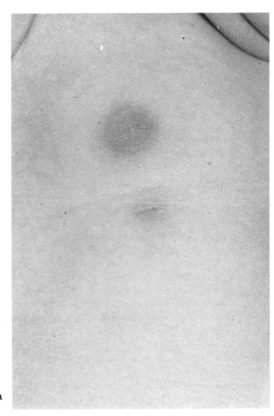

85. Supernumerary nipple in a newborn

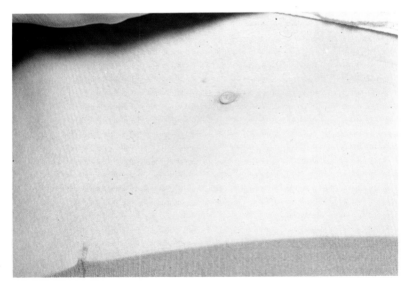

86. A supernumerary nipple in a mother near term demonstrating the absence of glandular tissue

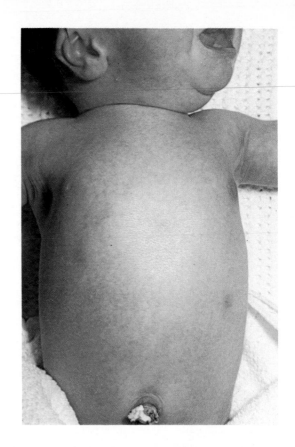

87. Multiple supernumerary nipples

88-91

Umbilicus cutis

Umbilicus amnioticus

If the skin portion of the navel encroaches unduly on the cord – umbilicus cutis (88) – this can leave an unsightly protusion which will require cosmetic surgery later. Contrariwise, the amniotic portion may encroach on the skin of the abdomen – umbilicus amnioticus (89); this is less common and the small para-umbilical hernia which sometimes remains is usually trivial. Para-umbilical hernia is more often associated with a normal navel (90); there may be evidence of Rectus diastasis which is obvious when the intra-abdominal pressure is raised. The cord is inspected in the delivery room – a single artery (91) may be the indicator of unsuspected internal malformation.

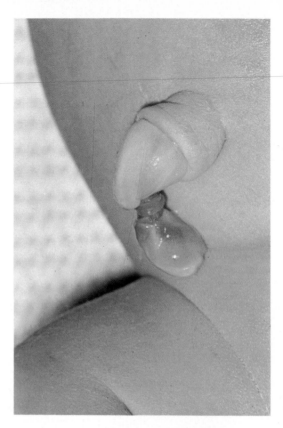

88. Umbilicus cutis

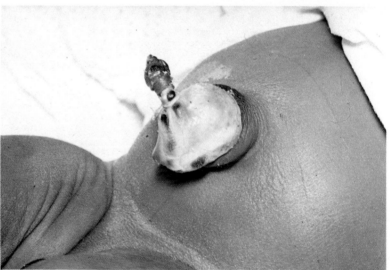

89. Umbilicus amnioticus

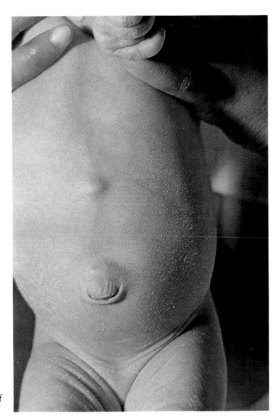

90. Paraumbilical hernia and hernia of linea alba

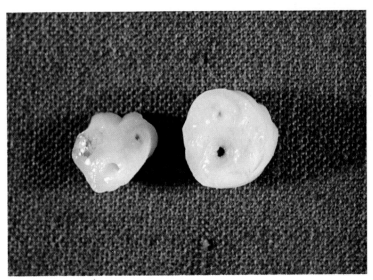

91. Single umbilical artery

Section two

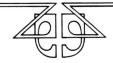

Low-birth-weight babies

The low-birth-weight baby is the 'premature' baby of former years. Today this and some other definitions have been sensibly superseded, but assessment and management are still founded on the basic concepts of 'immaturity', 'dysmaturity' and 'postmaturity'. The quality of survival has improved for many small babies but a number of the very smallest, who in the past would have succumbed, today survive only to inherit some of the old problems. Ultimately, preventive medicine would offer the best prospect of help, if it could ensure normal intrauterine nutrition and bring gestation safely to term.

The old definition of prematurity was a baby weighing 2500g. or less at birth. Such a baby would now be classified as a low-birth-weight child. This figure of 2500g. is the lower limit of the normal range of fetal weight at full term (280 postmenstrual days) in the developed countries of the 1930's (Diagram A), and the metric figure coincided conveniently with the Imperial $5\frac{1}{2}$lb. It was anomalous that a measure of time ('prematurity') should be qualified by a measure of weight, while important factors such as race, sex, rank and social class were disregarded. In any case, the additional risk incurred by the baby was very small where the birth weight exceeded about 1750g. The absurdity of the definition was emphasised by many maternal variables. It gave the healthy North American Negro female twice the 'prematurity' rate of her white cousin , and in any group of women fetal growth can vary significantly between gestations at sea level and those occurring at high altitudes. A comparison between the unqualified statement of birth weight 2500g. and the Caucasian norm (Diagram B) shows that the weight would lie within the normal range at 30-40 weeks' gestation but be classified as fetal malnutrition because the fetus is underweight after 40 weeks or overweight before 30 weeks!

It was always appreciated, however, that there existed two significantly different populations of small babies – those who were born too soon, and those who were 'dysmature' because of prenatal malnutrition. By agreement reached through the World Health Organisation it is internationally accepted that babies born too soon are called pre-term if they are born before 37 completed weeks of postmenstrual gestation (Diagram C), while 'dysmature' babies, called small-for-dates, are defined as those with a birth weight at or below the lower limit of the normal range for any gestational age (Diagram D). It would be logical to say 'light-for-dates' when the weight is below the lower limit of normal, but despite the purists' activities on nomenclature committees this expression has failed to achieve currency. The combination of pre-term and small-for-dates is easily defined on paper (Diagram E), although the clinician may not always intend these precise criteria when he speaks.

1-3

One cannot usually say with confidence that any particular baby's weight problem arises exclusively from shortness of gestation or smallness-for-dates. This is because, in common conditions like toxaemia, intrauterine malnutrition from poor placental function is compounded by early induction of labour. Logically one could surmise that the baby weighing 2500g. born at 35 weeks had been doing perfectly well until immediately before his untimely birth, whereas a baby weighing 2500g. at 40 weeks had been in trouble for some time, in some instances from the time of conception. Here the question of placental function is most germane. In the baby born at 35 weeks it would probably be normal, while in the 40-week baby it would commonly be deficient. This crucial difference is well emphasised where there is dissimilar growth in twins (Illustrations 1, 2, 3: the survivor had the better placental half and weighed 1275g. against the other's 600g.).

When low birth weight is recorded, the immediate problem for the clinician is to assess the baby's maturity so that he may know whether the weight is appropriate to the estimated gestational age. There are two main lines of clinical approach to this problem. One employs a scoring system based mainly on the physical properties of the skin and its appendages together with the sexual characteristics. The other is to assess the level to which certain postural, tonic and reflex phenomena have developed.

If smallness-for-dates is diagnosed a further problem arises. This is to try to recognise the cause and duration of the antecedent intrauterine failure to thrive. The problem bears a crude resemblance to some classical causes of failure to thrive which bring a six-month-old infant to the clinic (Diagram F); the neonatal problem is similar (Diagram G) in that it is necessary to know whether the failure to thrive in utero arose from fairly recent or from long-standing troubles.

Finally, we have to deal with the special situation where the baby may not be of low birth weight technically but has many of the characteristics of the small-for-dates baby and faces similar problems. Formerly known as 'postmature', this baby is now called post-term, and is defined as a baby born after more than 41 weeks of completed postmenstrual gestation.

Diagram A

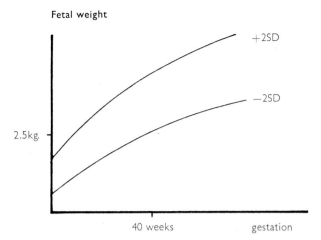

Fetal weight

+2SD

−2SD

2.5kg.

40 weeks   gestation

Diagram B

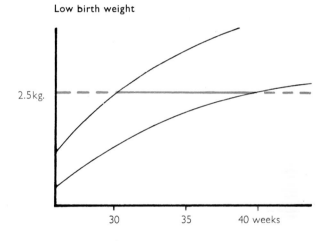

Low birth weight

2.5kg.

30   35   40 weeks

Diagram C

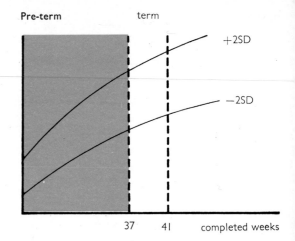

Diagram D

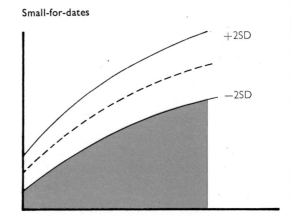

Diagram E

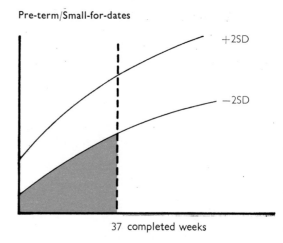

Diagram F

Failure to thrive (1)

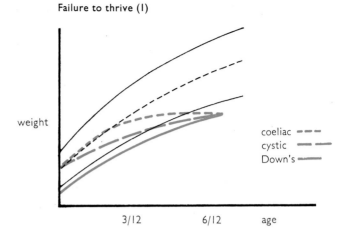

weight

coeliac - - -
cystic ━ ━
Down's ━━━

3/12   6/12   age

Diagram G

Failure to thrive (2)

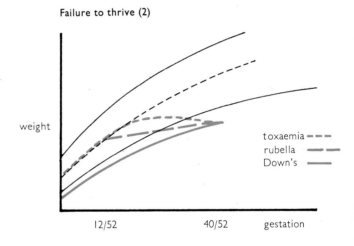

weight

toxaemia - - -
rubella ━ ━
Down's ━━━

12/52   40/52   gestation

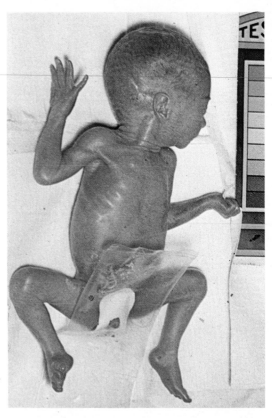

1, 2. Dissimilar growth in twins and the rich red ('boiled lobster') colour of the skin which is deeper than the *erythema neonatorum* seen at term

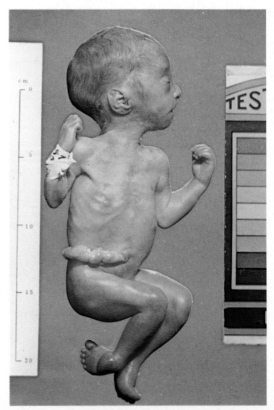

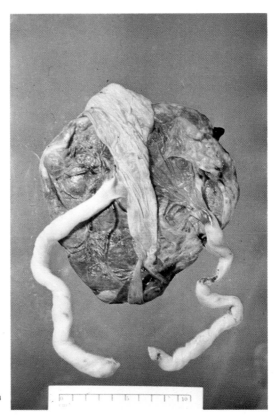

3. The placenta of the twins shown in
plates 1 and 2

1, 4-7	Body proportions	The relatively large head (1, 4, 5) is free from moulding and signs of intrauterine compression; the thoracic volume is small and the abdomen is usually prominent (4, 5) – although it may be flat (6, 7) – and the limbs are short in relation to the crown-rump length (4). This is in contrast with the even cylindrical contour at term when the head, chest and abdominal circumferences approximate to each other.
8, 9		At birth the fontanelles are small and the sutures narrow, but they soon gape under normal tension as the brain's growth-rate transiently outstrips that of the skull. The pre-term baby's abdominal prominence often persists for months (8) and preponderant recumbence in one lateral position may result in a mildly skew head (9).
10-13	Posture and movement	The dominant posture is one of deflexion with the limbs hardly supported off the underlying surface (10, 11), since the baby has escaped the effects of intrauterine compression at term and the underdeveloped muscle masses are weak and tone is low. It is his 'position of ease'. If a term infant adopts this posture in a good state of arousal it is called the 'frog position' and is a sign of illness (12: heart failure; 13: infant of diabetic mother).
14-18		If there is marked extension of the limbs, the resultant sprawled posture has the serene and sybaritic quality of sunbathing (14). The suggestion of relaxation may be heightened by frequent luxurious yawning (15, 16). The limbs often adopt the asymmetrical tonic neck posture (17) and this is more likely to be physiologically reversed (18) than in the term infant.
19		The baby rarely turns his head spontaneously from side to side. The weight and volume of the head are too much for the puny neck muscles to move it across the midline (19).
5, 10, 14, 15		The hands are open much of the time as part of the general deflexion (5, 10, 14, 15) and some crude movements of digital opposition may be seen.

11, 19, 20		Respiratory movement is mainly diaphragmatic because the intercostal muscles act weakly and mild recession of the sternum and costal margin is normal (11, 19, 20). Through the thin abdominal wall the movements of intestinal loops are readily visible (20).
1, 11, 18, 21-26	The skin	The appearance is usually shiny (21) especially in areas of mild oedema (11) or it may become wrinkled (18). The fine texture, combined with the paucity of subcutaneous fat, gives a transparent quality and subcutaneous vessels readily show through (22). Lanugo hair is often profuse (23, 24, 25). Soon after birth a rich red colour may develop (1), deeper than the *erythema neonatorum* seen at term. A little oedema is usual by the end of the first day (11), especially in the lower limbs; it may be aggravated and prolonged if the baby's immature kidneys cannot meet the extra solute load imposed by some artificial.milk formulas (26).
4, 20		The ear cartilage is deficient and soft. Consequently the pinna does not spring back readily if it has been pressed down (4, 20). On release it remains crumpled against the side of the head.
27, 28		Physiological jaundice is of slightly later onset than in the term infant, but it becomes more pronounced (27: bilirubin 12, 9, 13 mg. %) and is of longer duration (28: 2 weeks).
		In contrast with the skin at term, there is little or no vernix, desquamation is uncommon, *erythema toxicum* is rare, and the variegated pattern of dermatoglyphic creases is less well developed, especially on the sole of the foot.
29-31	Sexual characteristics	The clitoris is relatively large and this appearance is enhanced by vulval gaping due to separation of the labia majora and minora (29) sometimes causing intersex to be mistakenly suspected (30). Varying degrees of incomplete descent of the testicles occur (31).
22		The areola is flat and may be difficult to differentiate from the surrounding skin. The nipple itself may be hardly visible (22).

Transplacental hormonal effects such as mucoid vaginal secretion, withdrawal bleeding, breast hypertrophy and 'witch's milk' secretion are extremely unlikely; it is probable that they occur only in the term infant.

32-42 Physical vulnerability

The reason for this is the structural and functional immaturity of tissues and organs. The lungs may fail to expand under the poor respiratory effort, their appearance is fleshy and airless in atelectasis (32), and they sink in water (33). Even a well-inflated lung shows petechiae caused by rupture of the delicate capillaries (34). Pneumothorax may occur (35), or expansion may be incomplete, leading to respiratory distress (36), for example from hyaline membrane disease when the alveolar lining is deficient in its surfactant content. There is no great liability to haemorrhagic disease from prothrombin deficiency but fragile small vessels may rupture in various sites such as the brain substance (37), its ventricles (38) or meninges (39, 40), the bowel wall (41) or the endocardium (42: 'blood cyst' on mitral cusp). This is probably aggravated by anoxia.

36, 43

The delicate vessels also suffer from the ministrations of the medical attendant, whether these are forceful as in breech extraction (43) or gentle as in electrocardiography (36). On the other hand, the pre-term baby is relatively free from certain forms of obstetric trauma such as nerve palsies, fractures and cephalhaematoma.

44

Some tissues have a peculiar chemical vulnerability, the extrapyramidal portion of the nervous system will be poisoned by levels of unconjugated bilirubin that a bigger baby could withstand; this can lead to kernicterus. A high concentration of oxygen can damage the eye, causing retrolental fibroplasia (44).

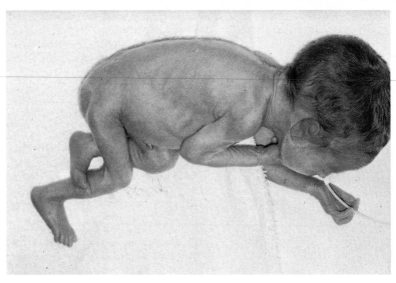

4. Body proportions. Deficient and soft
ear cartilage

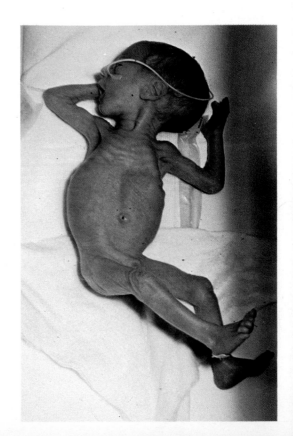

5. Body proportions and hand posture

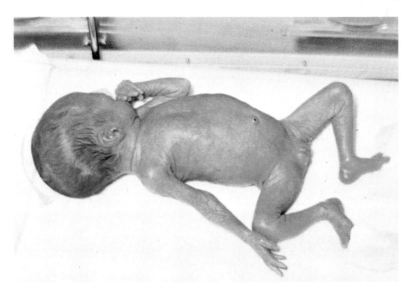

6. The less usual flat abdomen

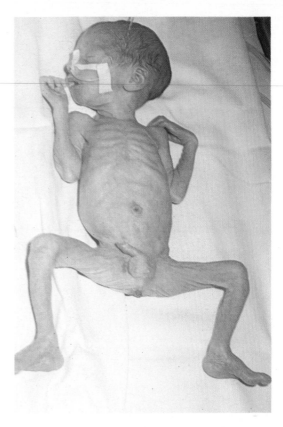

7. The less usual flat abdomen

8. Persistent abdominal prominence
after several months

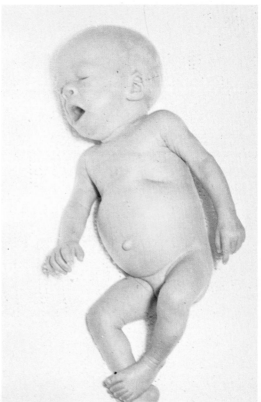

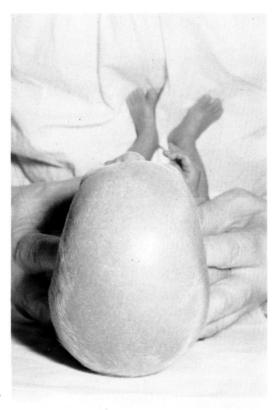

9. Mildly skew head after lying pre-dominently in one lateral position

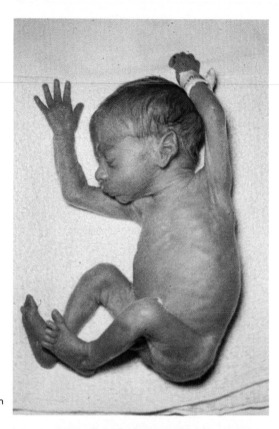

10. The dominant posture of deflexion with open hands

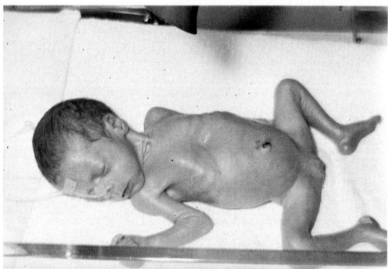

11. The dominant posture. Mild oedema and shiny skin. Mild recession of the sternum and costal margin

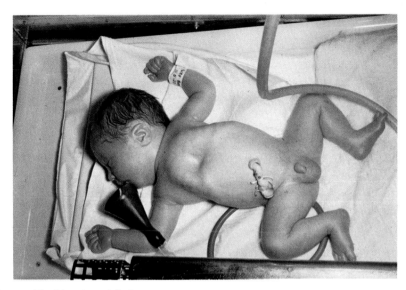

12. The 'frog position' in a term infant
with heart failure

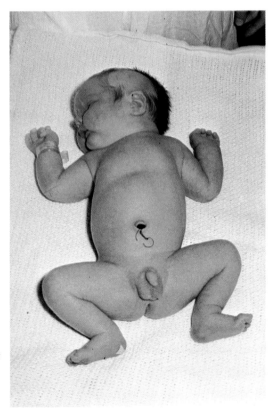

13. The 'frog position' in a term infant of
a diabetic mother

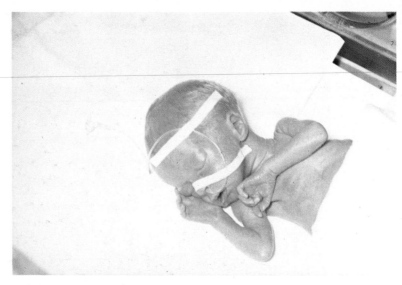

14. Movements of digital opposition

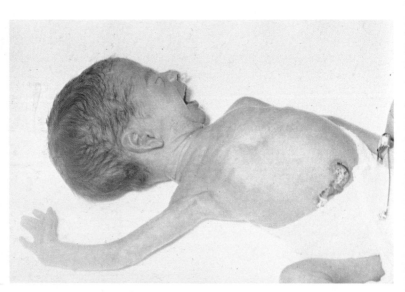

15. Luxurious yawning and open hand

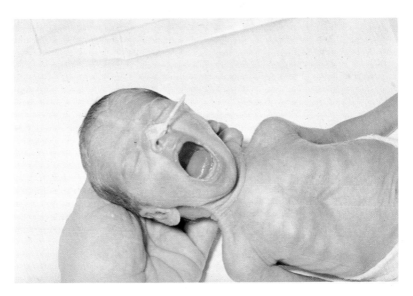

16. Yawning

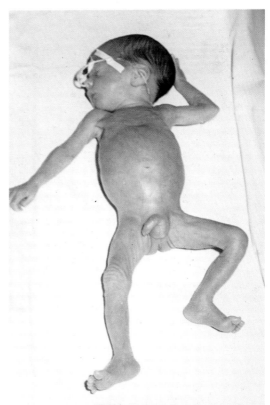

17. Relaxed asymmetrical tonic neck posture

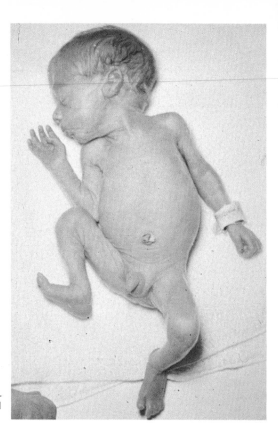

18. Physiologically reversed asymmetrical tonic neck posture. Wrinkled
skin

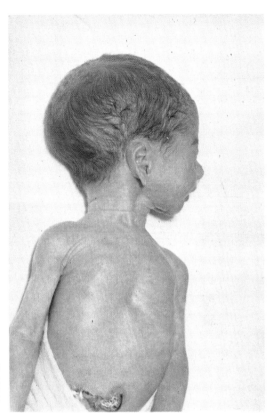

19. The puny neck muscles are unable to move the head from side to side. Mild recession of the sternum and costal margin in the mainly diaphragmatic respiration

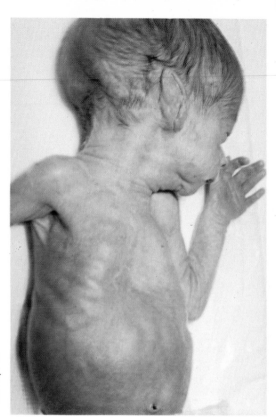

20. Mild recession of the sternum and costal margin in the mainly diaphragmatic respiration. Movements of intestinal loops readily visible through the thin abdominal wall. Deficient and soft ear cartilage

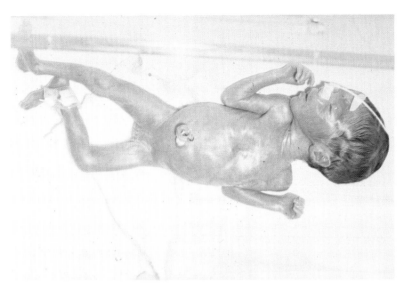

21. Shiny skin

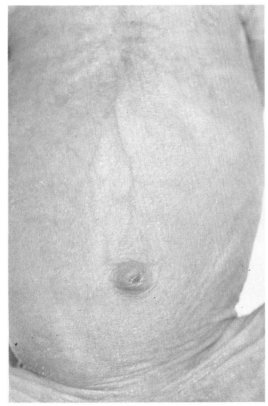

22. Transparent quality of the skin. The nipple is barely visible

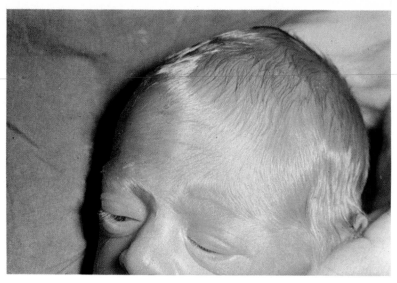

23. Profuse lanugo hair

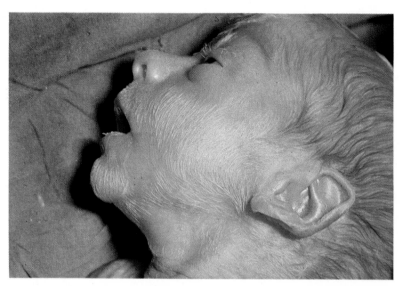

24. Profuse lanugo hair

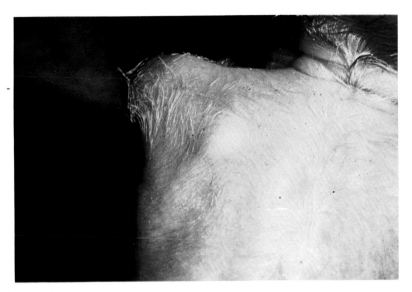

25. Profuse lanugo hair

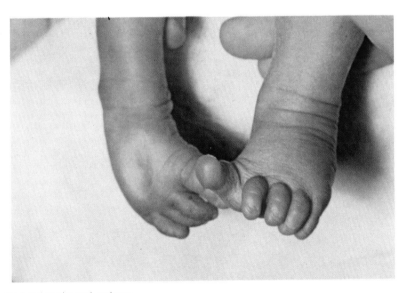

26. Aggravated and prolonged oedema
when the immature kidneys cannot cope
with some artificial milk formulas

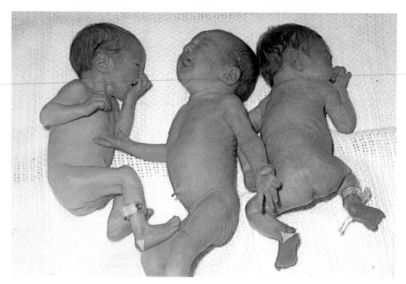

27. Physiological jaundice of later onset and more pronounced than in the term infant

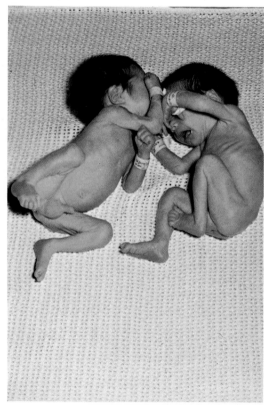

28. Physiological jaundice of two weeks duration

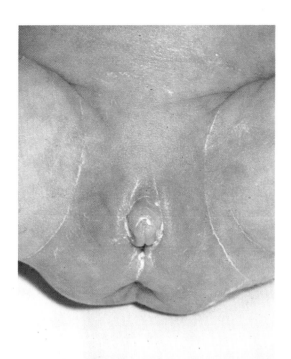

29. Genitalia of the female pre-term
infant

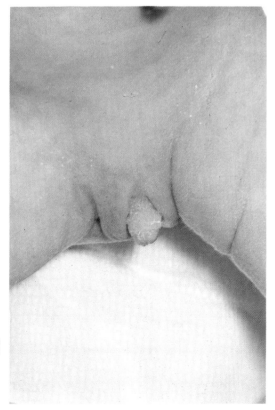

30. The relatively large size of the
clitoris in the pre-term infant may lead
to a mistaken diagnosis of intersex

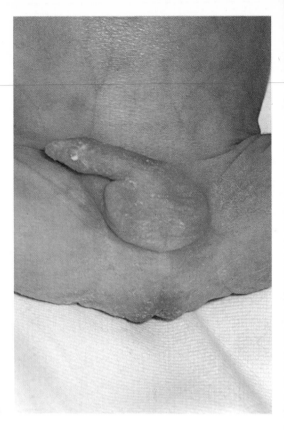

31. Incomplete descent of the testicles

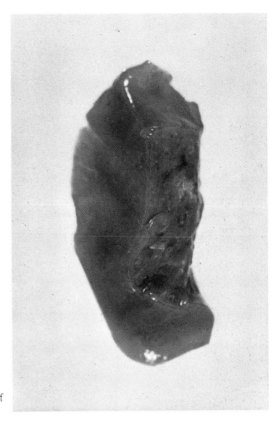

32. Fleshy and airless appearance of the lungs in atelectasis

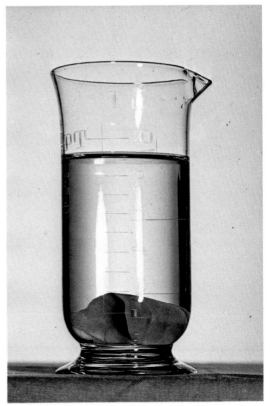

33. The lung in plate 32 sinks in water

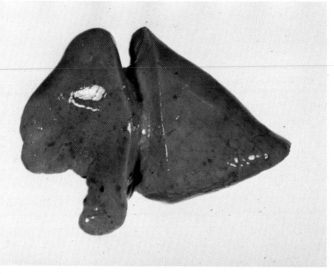

34. Petechiae in a well-inflated lung

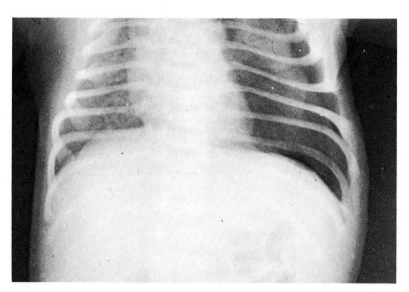

35. Pneumothorax

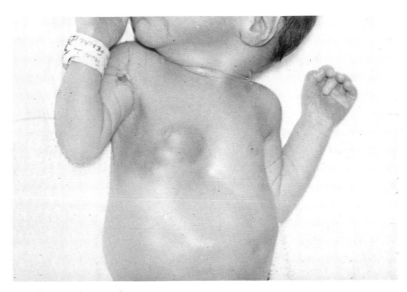

36. Respiratory distress due to incomplete expansion. Damage to delicate skin vessels from a procedure as gentle as electrocardiography

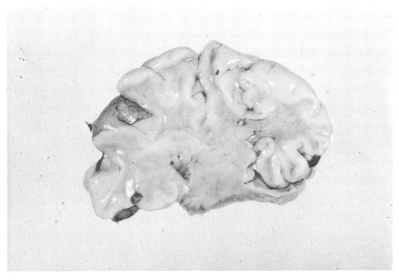

37. Rupture of fragile small vessels in the brain

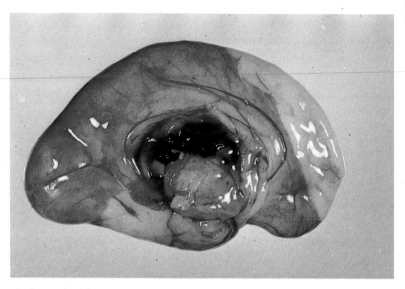

38. Intraventricular cerebral haemorrhage

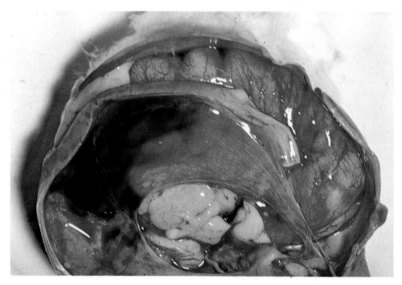

39. Rupture of fragile vessels in the falx

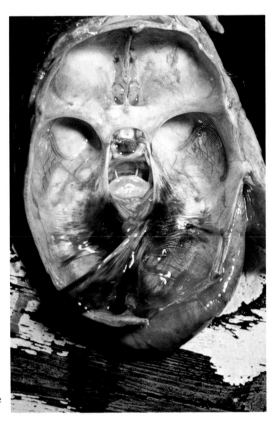

40. Rupture of fragile vessels in the tentorium

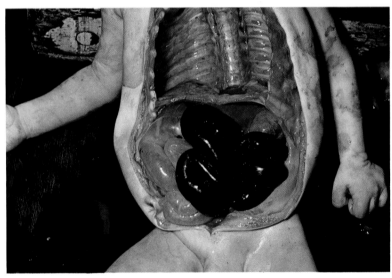

41. Rupture of vessels in the bowel wall

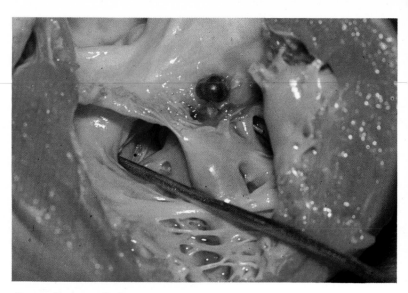

42. 'Blood cyst' on a mitral cusp. Probe
in ventricular septal defect

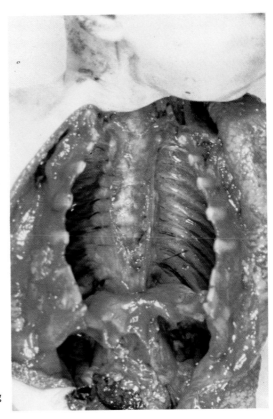

43. Adrenal haemorrhage following
breech extraction

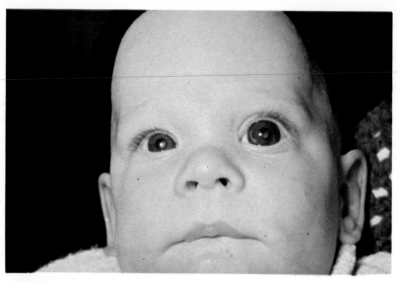

44. Retrolental fibroplasia due to high
oxygen concentration

45, 46

The baby's appearance, proportions and behaviour are closer to those of the term infant than at the mean gestational age normally appropriate to his birth weight (45: 2200g., 38 weeks estimated gestation). First one must exclude the possibility of congenital abnormalities such as major malformation (or of acquired embryopathy for example from fetal rubella), where there is a high risk, of the order of 5-15 per cent. What one usually sees is only the signs of protein-energy deprivation: the baby is relatively long and thin and often has meconium staining because of fetal distress. The placenta should be examined as it is often the seat of trouble (46).

Unless such babies are ill, they feed more competently than their pre-term equivalent, their physiological weight loss is slight, and they quickly return to birth weight. There is less tendency to physiological jaundice.

47-49

It is often necessary to carry out resuscitation because the birth process commonly results in asphyxia and acidosis, perhaps with hypoglycaemia. A good pharyngeal suckout is mandatory if the liquor or skin is meconium stained, and the gastric contents should be aspirated (47). This is to prevent massive meconium aspiration (48), which causes severe pneumonitis. There is an increased risk of pneumonia in these babies (49); the low gamma-globulin level in the blood may be a predisposing factor.

50, 51

There is one peculiar area of physical vulnerability; respiratory difficulty may be associated with the clinical and radiological signs of a pneumonia (50), which will not respond to treatment and the child may prove to have massive intrapulmonary haemorrhage (51). The reduced frequency of this condition in recent years probably reflects the measures taken to prevent hypothermia and hypoglycaemia which are its usual concomitants.

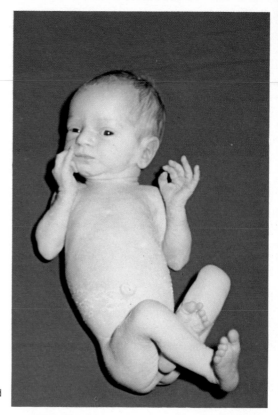

45. A baby of 38 weeks estimated gestation weighing 2,200 g

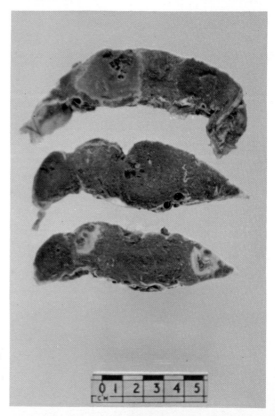

46. Macroscopic appearance of the placenta of the baby in plate 45

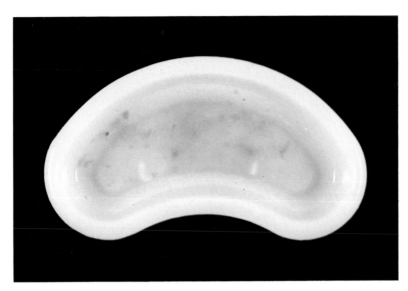

47. Aspirated gastric contents

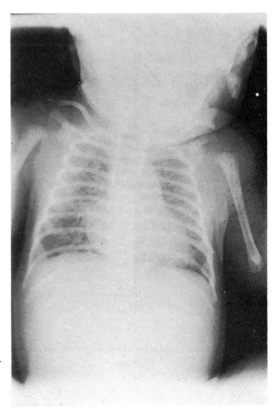

48. Massive   meconium   aspiration.
Meconium pneumonitis

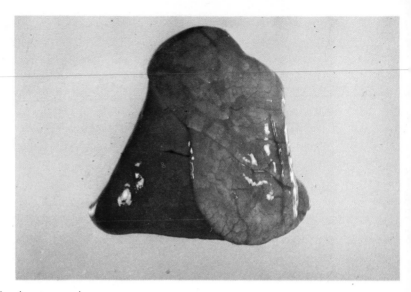

49. Lung showing pneumonia

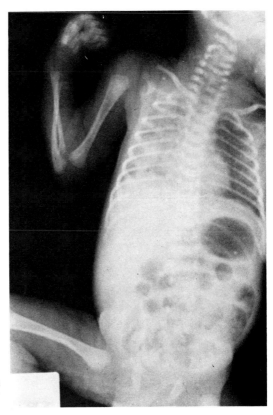

50. Radiological signs of pneumonia due to massive intrapulmonary haemorrhage

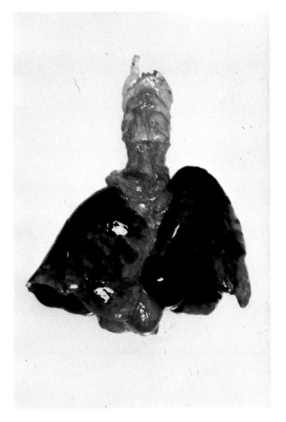

51. Lungs from the baby in plate 50

The post-term baby

After term, the effectiveness with which the placenta functions decreases and the volume of liquor diminishes – but the baby's linear growth proceeds fairly well. A virtual state of siege begins, in which the increasingly cramped and compressed baby has to deal with protein-energy malnutrition by consuming his own energy stores. This process takes place under the disadvantage of increasing hypoxia, perhaps until distress induces the passage of meconium to secure an assisted delivery.

52-59, 61, 63

The baby is long and skinny (52) and has a hard skull because the sutures have started to fuse; the skin is loose and dry like parchment, without lanugo hair and the hands are like a washerwoman's (61, 63). If there is meconium staining (53) a good suckout of the upper air passages is required and the stomach should be emptied. After a few days there is extensive cracking and peeling (54, 55, 56, 57, 58). The cranial hair may be overgrown and the fingernails long (59). The baby looks and behaves as if he had already lived out the first post-term weeks; the skin is white and does not develop *erythema neonatorum* or *erythema toxicum*. The baby is wakeful and if he has had an easy delivery his primitive reflex responses are lively.

60-63

If there is neurological disturbance after a difficult delivery the baby may be jittery and overactive. This may lead to the cracking of his frail skin by rubbing (60) or scratching with his long fingernails (61). Cephalhaematoma may result from birth trauma to the hard unyielding skull (62). Vomiting is common, with the hazard of aspiration and the special risk of meconium pneumonitis; there is also a risk of vomit burn from the physiologically strong neonatal gastric juice (63).

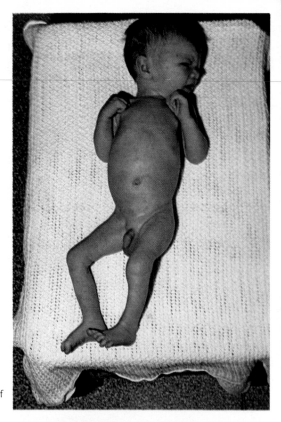

52. The long and skinny appearance of the post-term baby

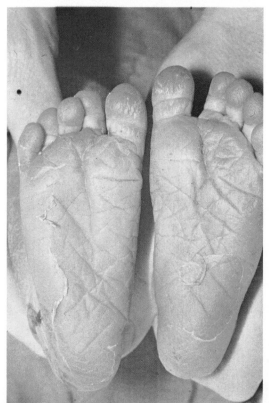

53. Meconium staining and peeling of the skin

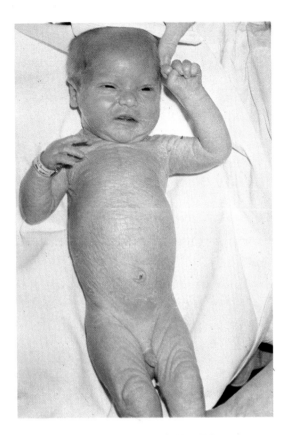

54. Extensive cracking of the skin

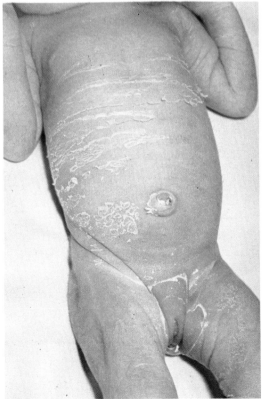

55. Extensive peeling of the skin

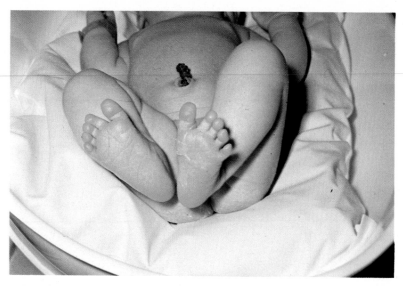

56. Peeling of the skin

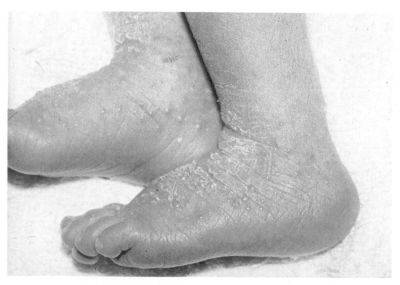

57. Cracking and peeling of the skin

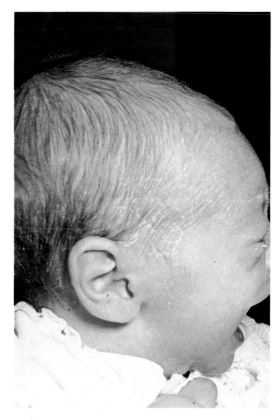

58. Peeling of the skin

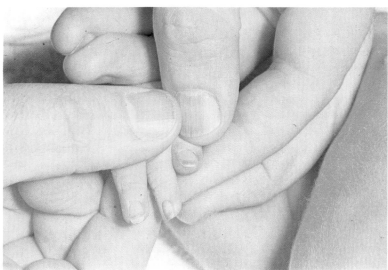

59. Long fingernails

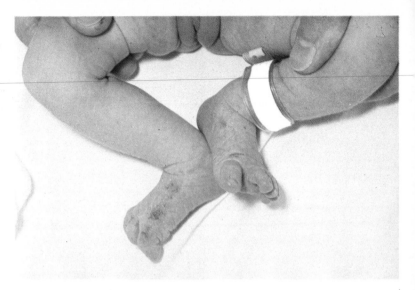

60. Skin damage from rubbing in an
overactive baby after a difficult delivery

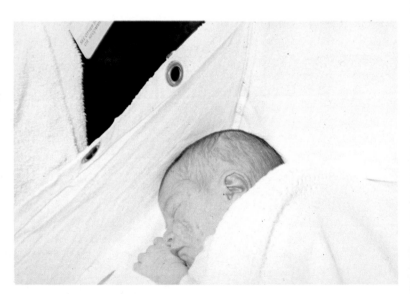

61. 'Washerwoman's hands'. Facial
scratches from the long fingernails

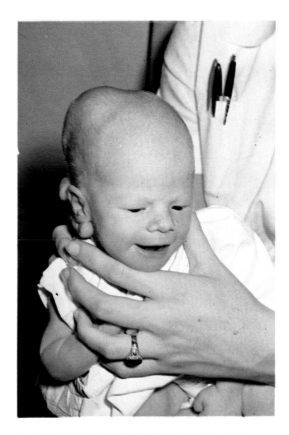

62. Cephalhaematoma

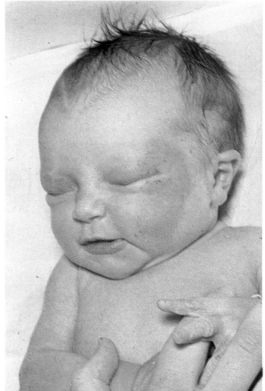

63. 'Washerwoman's hands'. Vomit burn from physiologically strong neonatal gastric juices

Section three

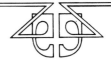

Trauma

Introduction

Improving standards of obstetric care have reduced the severe traumatic effects of difficult delivery. One happy result is that certain forms of intranatally determined cerebral palsy have become less common. On the other hand, more low-birth-weight babies survive and they are especially vulnerable. The universal application of screening tests involving physical interference has also led inevitably to an increase in minor traumatic phenomena in the nursery.

The subject can be taken in sequence from intrauterine life through spontaneous delivery and on to the hazards that a baby can face from the helping efforts of the obstetrician, midwife or paediatrician (apart from the damage which babies sometimes inflict on themselves or which is caused by members of the family). Finally, a look will be taken at some of the pitfalls which can lead to mistaken diagnosis.

Intrauterine

1, 2

Compressional effects on the baby's head and neck are common, and usually trivial. If, however, ear-to-shoulder compression is severe, for example in the post-term baby, a 'sternomastoid tumour' may develop after a couple of weeks (1) and may on rare occasions be bilateral (2: after breech). Facial palsy can also result from such compression, or from the pressure of a foot on the nerve in a breech baby with extended legs.

3-5

Pressure over a well-padded area with underlying bony structures may cause subcutaneous fat necrosis (3, 4). Closer to term, the frenzied movements of fetal distress may inflict scratches (5) particularly if the baby is equipped with long fingernails due to post-maturity.

6-8

Diagnostic and therapeutic amniocentesis (6) is a new hazard for an increasing number of babies. Some rare phenomena such as congenital 'gangrene' (7) have the appearance of traumatic necrosis, but the mechanism is not fully understood. Congenital partial thickness skin defects are similar in appearance (8); amniotic adhesions when present are probably secondary and not causative.

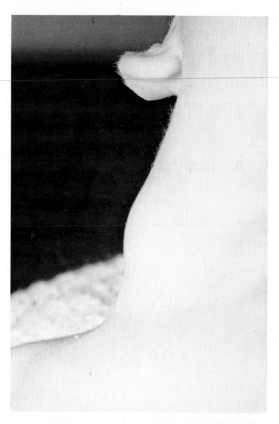

1. Sternomastoid tumour at two weeks of age

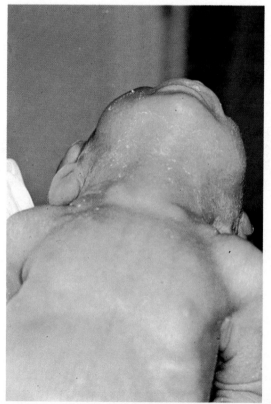

2. Bilateral sternomastoid tumour after breech presentation

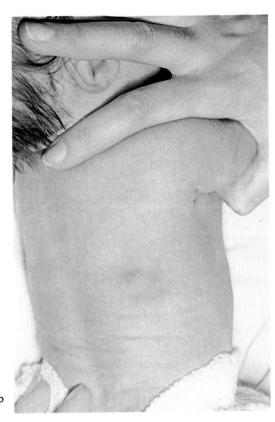

3. Subcutaneous fat necrosis due to pressure

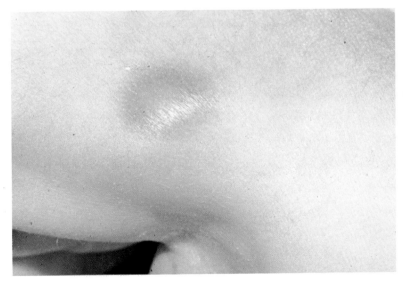

4. Subcutaneous fat necrosis due to pressure

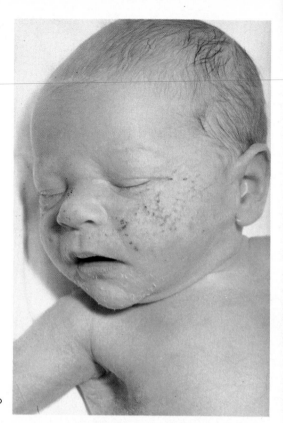

5. Facial scratches inflicted in utero by the movements of fetal distress

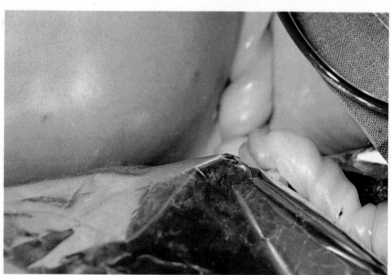

6. Lesions inflicted during intrauterine transfusion

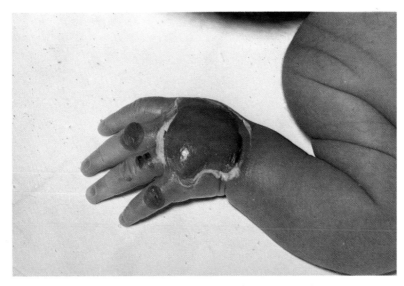

7. Congenital 'gangrene'

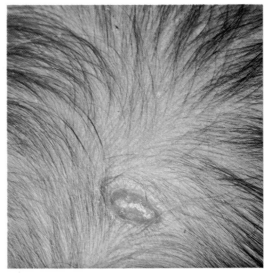

8. Congenital partial thickness skin defect of the scalp

9-16

In a vertex presentation, if the second stage is precipitate or obstructed, petechial haemorrhages (9) may occur. If the mother contributes by bearing down before the cervix is fully dilated, she herself may suffer something similar (10). Malpresentation of face (11) or brow (12) causes bruising and petechiae, and if the cord is tight round the neck the consequent mechanical purpura may be widespread (13). Haemorrhage is easily caused in the eyelids and conjunctivae (14). Intraorbital haemorrhage may result in proptosis (15) and as the blood tracks forward it is contained by the palpebral fascia and causes the clear-cut type of black eye (16) dear to the comic cartoonist; the blood may come from a linear fracture of the orbital plate of the frontal bone.

17

In low-birth-weight babies there is often haemorrhage or extravasation from small fragile intracranial vessels and sometimes a tentorial tear with greater trauma (17).

18-23,
45, 54

Delay in the second stage causes the presenting part to press through the partly-dilated cervix (18), whose constricting rim obstructs the return flow of venous blood and lymph from the scalp, leading to oedema. This is called *caput succedaneum* (19). Its distribution lies across suture lines (20) and, characteristically of oedema, it pits on pressure (19, 45, 54). Rarely, there may be blisters or a cervix mark (21). Since delivery relieves the causative obstruction, the swelling is maximal at birth and it goes away within a few days (Diagram A). In breech delivery, delay in the second stage results in similar oedema and bruising of the perineum, buttocks (22) and genitalia (23: a girl).

Diagram A

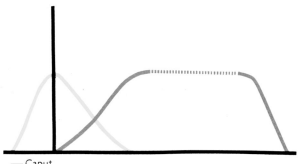

— Caput
■■■ Cephalhaematoma

19, 24-36

Caput is easily distinguishable from another traumatic swelling on the head, cephalhaematoma. This is a subpericranial collection of blood due to bleeding from a small fracture or vessel rupture (24a) at the time of birth. It is commonest after prolonged primigravid labour or forceps delivery, especially if the baby is post-term and suture fusion has made the skull hard and unyielding. In contrast with caput, the presence of cephalhaematoma is not apparent in the early hours after delivery but it grows slowly to its maximum size in the course of the next few days (Diagram A). It then remains static when the ooze of blood is stopped by clotting or vessel retraction or through the mechanical resistance of the elevated pericranium (24b). If it reaches a suture line, it is halted because the pericranium enters there (25a); this helps to distinguish it from caput especially when there is bilateral cephalhaematoma (26, 27, 28). Usually it is situated over the parietal bone (29) and the occipital region is the next most common site (30). It is easy to indent the liquefied blood-clot in the swelling with the tip of a finger. The blood-clot has a rubbery feel, and, on release of the pressure, springs out quickly without pitting. Cephalhaematoma persists for several weeks or months. It may then resolve quite rapidly unless extensive calcification or ossification has occurred (31). There is a diagnostic pitfall early on: the osteoblasts at the edge of the elevated pericranium survive to lay down new bone (25b), and form after a few days a ridge like a low volcano cone (25c, 33); this is sometimes mistaken for a depressed fracture. Distinction between the two relies upon the fact that the cephalhaematoma ridge is elevated so that the examining finger goes up and then down again before returning to the cranial surface (32a), whereas with depressed fracture there is a simple dip between the two levels (32b, 34). Jaundice frequently occurs with cephalhaematoma (35) as the blood breaks down, and liver function is often compromised by perinatal anoxia in these babies. In view of their mechanical origins it is not surprising that caput and cephalhaematoma often go together in a patient (19, 36). Both offer a breeding-ground for infection in devitalised tissue and should not be interfered with.

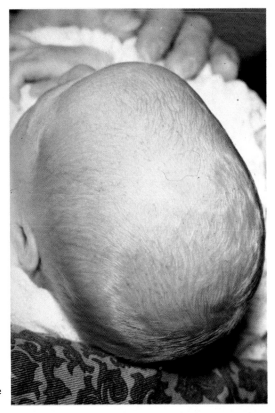

9. Petechial haemorrhages on the scalp of the infant

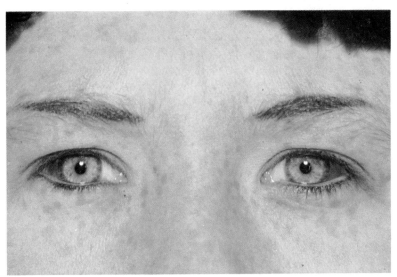

10. Subconjunctival haemorrhages in a mother

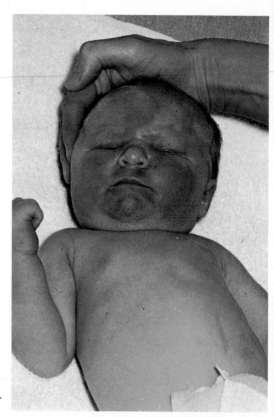

11. Bruising following face presentation

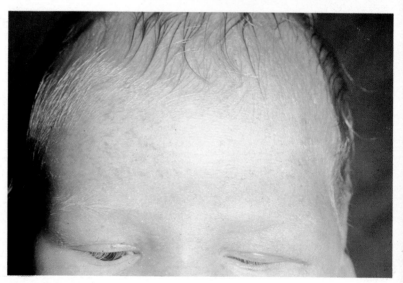

12. Petechiae following brow presentation

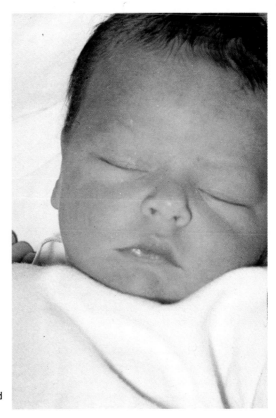

13. Mechanical purpura, cord around the neck

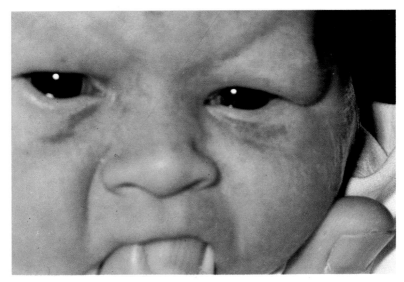

14. Haemorrhage in the eyelids and conjunctiva

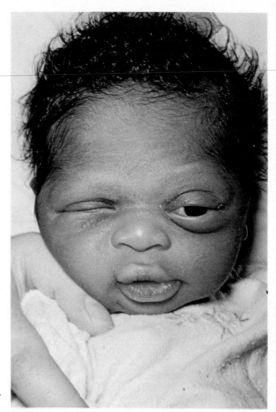

15. Protopsis, intraorbital haemorrhage

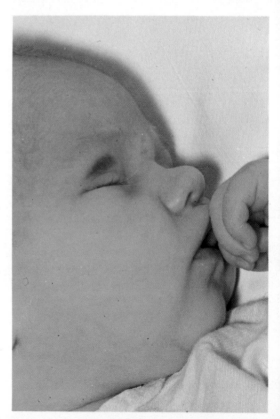

16. Black eye, intraorbital haemorrhage

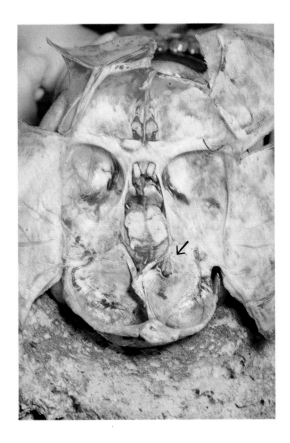

17. Tentorial tear

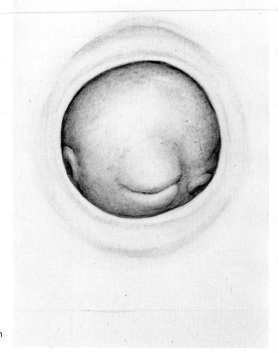

18. Presenting part pressing through
the partly dilated cervix

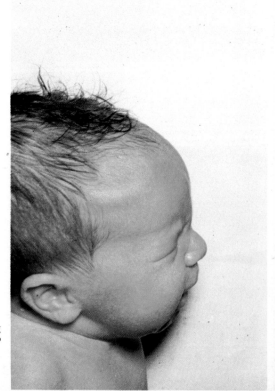

19. *Caput succedaneum* showing pitting
on pressure. Cephalhaematoma is also
present in this baby

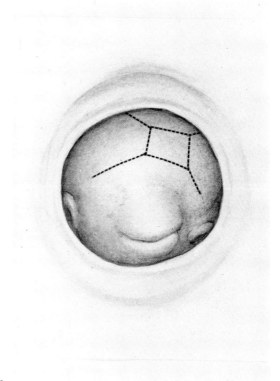

20. Distribution of oedema across suture lines in *caput succedaneum*

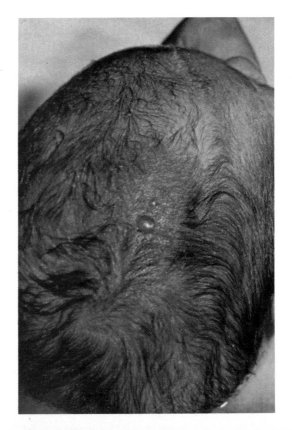

21. Blistering, 'cervix mark'

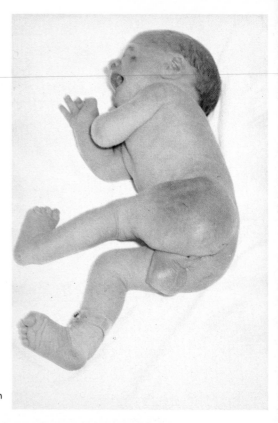

22. Bruising of the buttocks in breech delivery

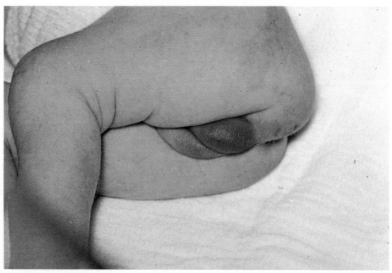

23. Oedema and bruising of the genitalia (a girl) in breech delivery

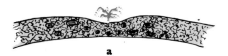

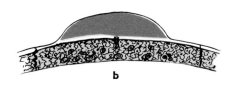

24. The gradual development of cephalhaematoma

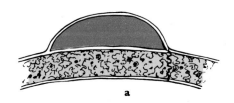

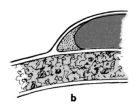

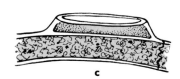

25. Cephalhaematoma halted at a suture line and cephalhaematoma rim like a low volcano cone

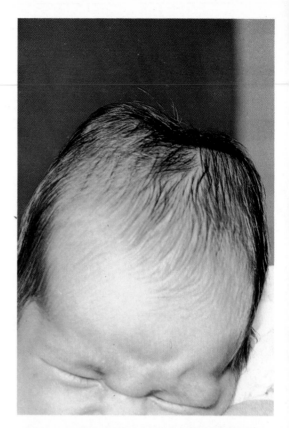

26. Bilateral cephalhaematoma

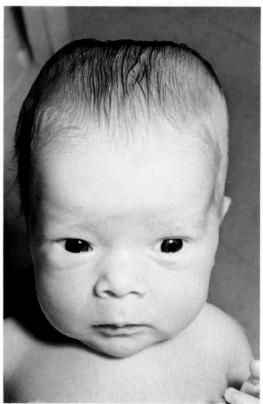

27. Bilateral cephalhaematoma

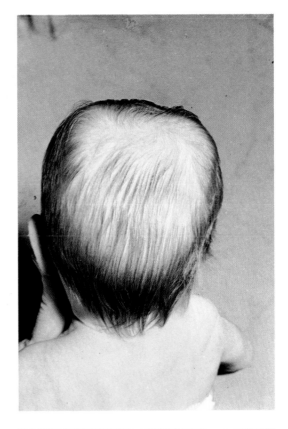

28. Bilateral cephalhaematoma

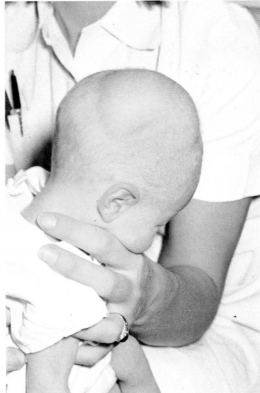

29. Cephalhaematoma over the parietal bone

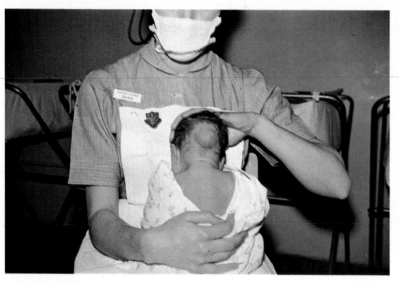

30. Cephalhaematoma   over   the
occipital bone

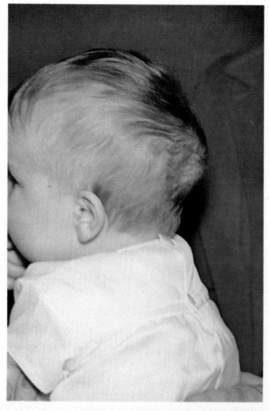

31. Persistent cephalhaematoma after
several months

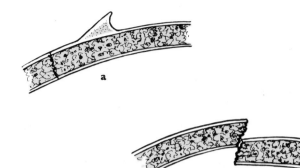

32. The distinction between cephalhaematoma rim and a depressed fracture

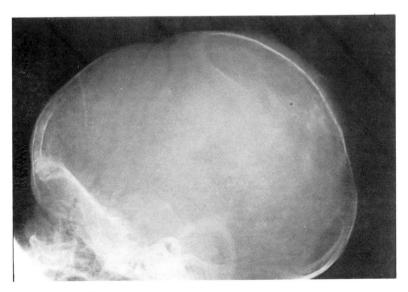

33. Cephalhaematoma rim on X-ray

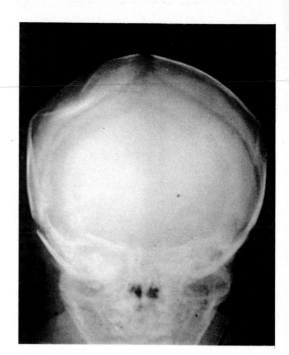

34. Depressed fracture

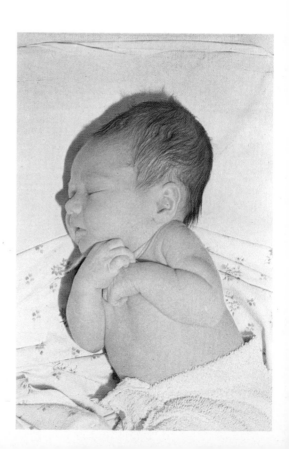

35. Jaundice with cephalhaematoma

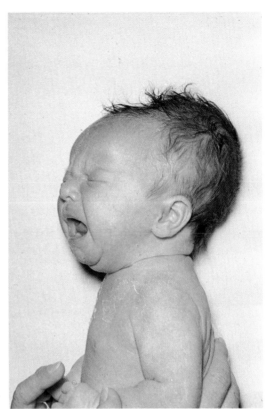

36. Concomitant caput and cephal-haematoma

37-40

The traumatic effects of intrapartum obstetric help arise from mechanical induction of labour, fetal sampling and operative, instrumental and assisted delivery. Artificial rupture of the membranes and fetal sampling result in small incised wounds – usually trivial – of the presenting part (37, 38, 39). In Caesarean section the site of the wound is more varied (40).

41-51

Forceps application causes bruises, ecchymoses and abrasions at a variety of sites (41, 42, 43, 44). This may lead to secondary infection if the skin is broken (45), subcutaneous fat necrosis (46), subconjunctival haemorrhage (47), facial palsy, which is usually transient (48) or fractured skull, either linear or depressed. Sometimes a permanent scar is caused (49) and in the unlikely event of facial paralysis persisting (50) there will be some degree of hemiatrophy (51).

52-54

Ventouse extraction applies vacuum suction to assist delivery when there is delay in the second stage. This may simply result in ecchymosis (52), but the baby often has caput which may be distorted into a 'chignon' (53), or the vulnerable skin may be blistered or lacerated (54), especially if the cup twists round to exert a shearing force on the boggy scalp tissue.

55-60

Fractures can result from manually-assisted delivery; the clavicle is the bone most affected (55). Fracture of the clavicle leads to a pseudoparesis of the upper limb. The swelling due to callus formation is not at its most apparent for a couple of weeks (56). The brachial plexus nerve elements may be harmed by traction; most often affected are the upper roots and the result of this is Erb's palsy (57: 'waiter accepting a tip'). If the lower roots are affected the result is Klumpke's palsy, which affects the small muscles of the hand and the palmar grasp reflex. If most of the roots are affected, a more severe brachial paralysis (58) is caused and the possibility of Horner's syndrome, or paralysis of the hemidiaphragm, should be considered. Incomplete recovery results in undergrowth of the limb (59). If congenital Horner's syndrome persists, the patient has heterochromia (60) caused by failure of secondary pigmentation to develop in the affected eye.

Breech extraction of the low-birth-weight baby runs the special additional hazards of adrenal haemorrhage, liver rupture or subcapsular haematoma.

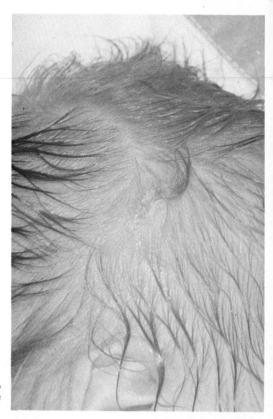

37. Small incised wound of the scalp following artificial rupture of the membranes

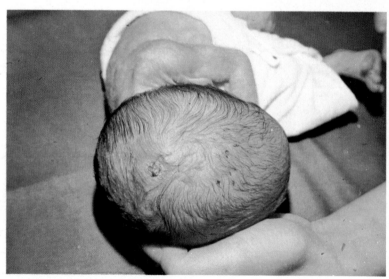

38. Small incised wound of the scalp following artificial rupture of the membranes

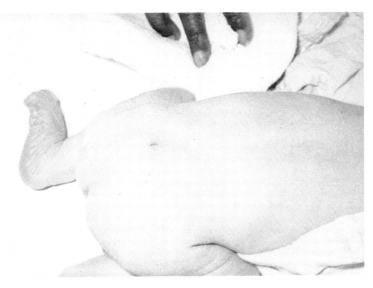

39. Small incised wound of the lower lumbar region following artificial rupture of the membranes

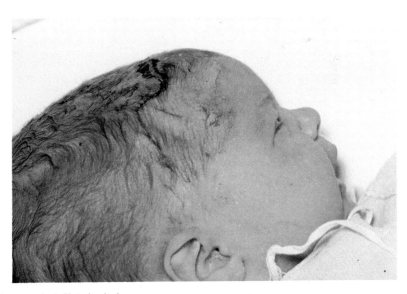

40. Incised wound inflicted during Cæsarean section

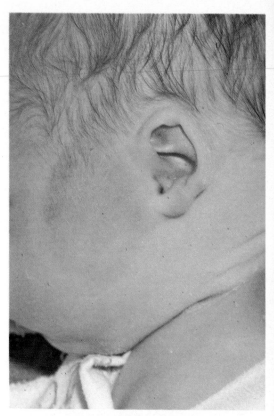

41. Trauma during forceps delivery

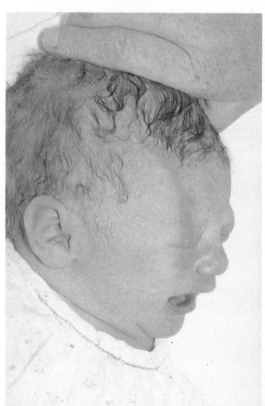

42. Trauma during forceps delivery

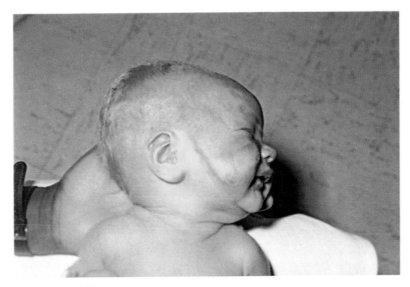

43. Trauma during forceps delivery

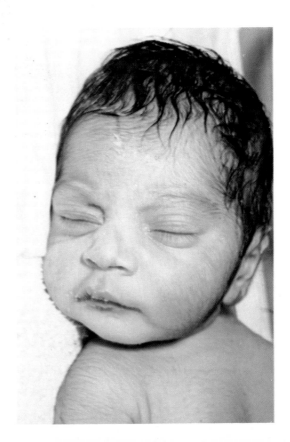

44. Trauma during forceps delivery

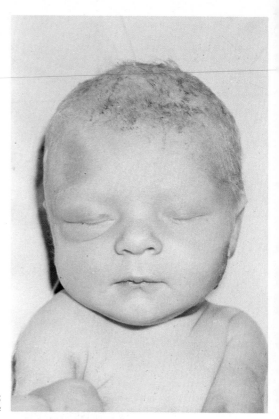

45. Secondary infection of broken skin;
caput succedaneum which pits on pressure

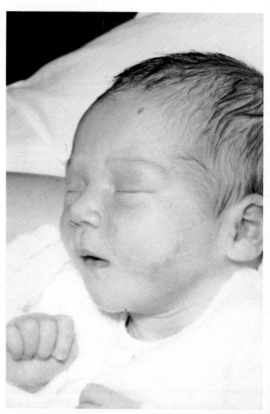

46. Subcutaneous fat necrosis following
trauma during forceps delivery

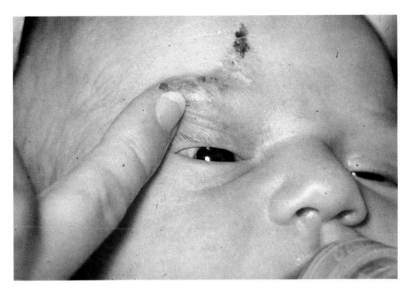

47. Subconjunctival haemorrhage
following forceps delivery

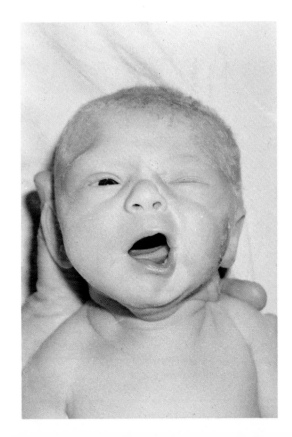

48. Transient facial palsy

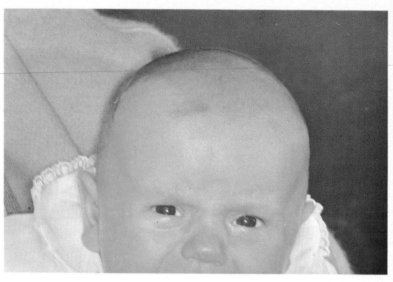

49. Permanent scarring

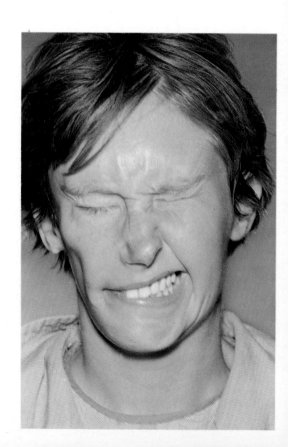

50. Permanent facial palsy

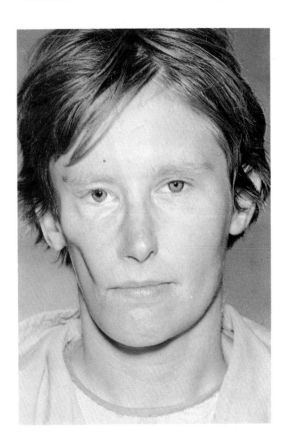

51. Hemiatrophy with facial paralysis

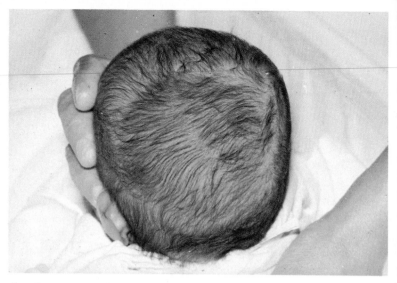

52. Ecchymosis due to ventouse extraction

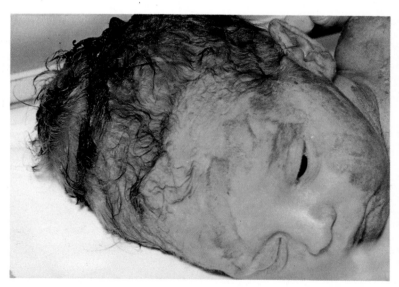

53. Caput distorted into a 'chignon' following ventouse extraction

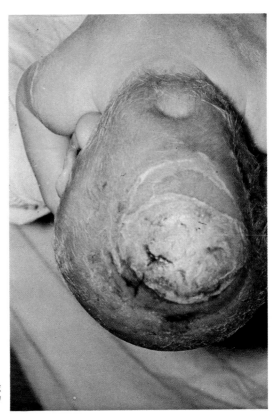

54. Laceration of the scalp during ventouse extraction; *caput succedaneum* which pits on pressure

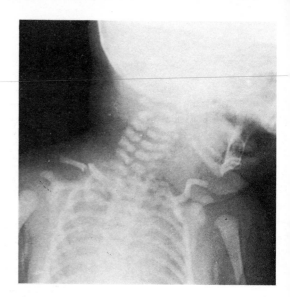

55. Fractured clavicle

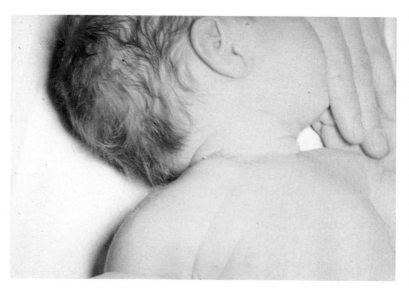

56. Swelling due to callus formation
after fracture of the clavicle

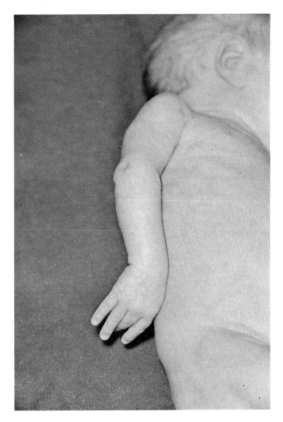

57. Erb's palsy following traction

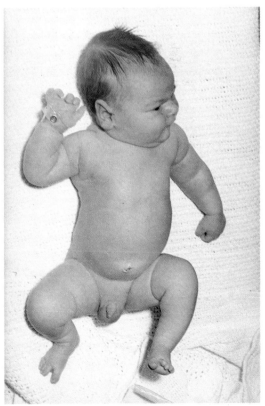

58. Brachial paralysis

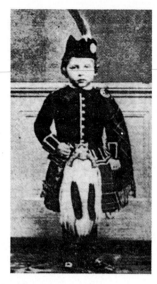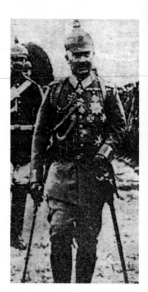

59. Undergrowth of the arm due to incomplete recovery from brachial paralysis

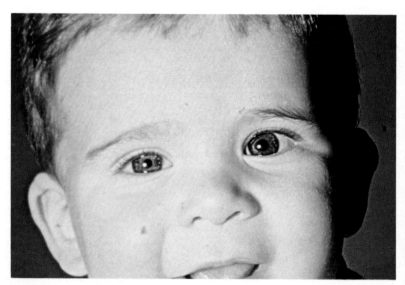

60. Heterochromia in congenital Horner's syndrome

Misadventure may occur early on, in hurriedly clamping the cord (61) or even in wrapping the baby or the mother (62: hot towel clip burn). Overtight swaddling can cause subcutaneous fat necrosis above the elbow from pressure of the contralateral knuckles (63); a little 'rosary' may be felt. If the heel has to be warmed for capillary blood collection, a miscalculation of the water temperature may cause scalding (64, 65). Necrosis can result from the intramuscular injection of substances intended for other routes (66) or from the use of inappropriate syringes (67). Sensitive skin reacts sometimes even to strapping applied to hold a dressing in place (68). Taking blood from the heel for sampling can also cause a mild, late traumatic effect (69).

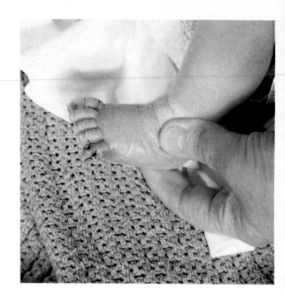

61. Mishap during cord clamping

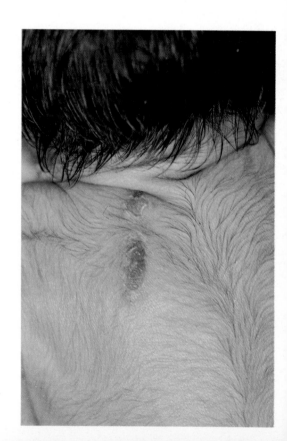

62. Hot towel clip burn

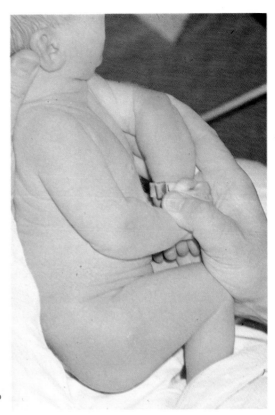

63. Subcutaneous fat necrosis due to
overtight swaddling

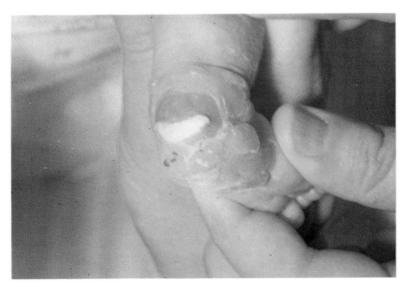

64. Scalding of the heel

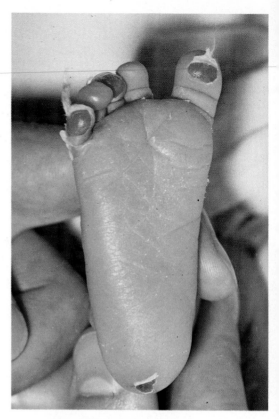

65. Scalding of the foot

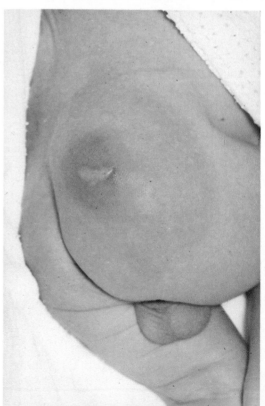

66. Necrosis due to intramuscular
injection of calcium solution

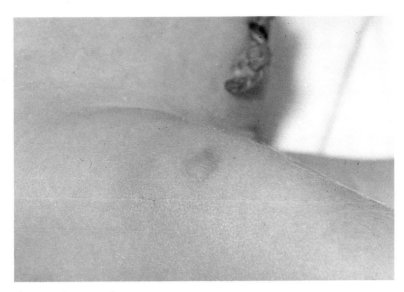

67. Trauma due to the use of an
inappropriate syringe

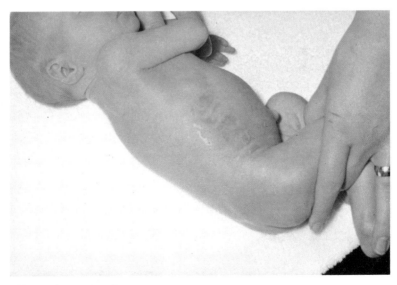

68. Sensitive skin reaction to strapping
to hold a dressing in place

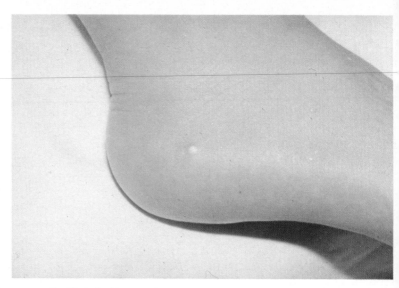

69. Mild, late traumatic effect of taking
blood from the heel

Paediatrician

70-76

In experienced hands, the routine examination of the baby in the nursery is quite safe. Very occasionally, however, the beginner may be so inept as to cause bony injury when he is testing hip stability or as he collects heelprick blood. However, the baby who needs help is delicate to start with; most of the investigative and therapeutic measures inherently involve traumatic hazards. Venepuncture can cause haemorrhage or thrombosis and necrosis (70), and even surgical emphysema (71). When the baby is ill, especially if he is of low-birth-weight, the simplest physical insult (72) may be too much for the fragile tissues (73). Some of the late effects of trauma may not be evident for months or years (74: site of subdural taps). Vaccination sites should be chosen on the upper limb because it is here that secondary infection is less likely (75) and the inflammatory swelling is more painful where the subcutaneous tissue is firmly tacked down (76).

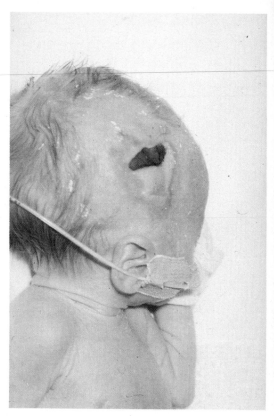

70. Thrombosis and necrosis following venepuncture

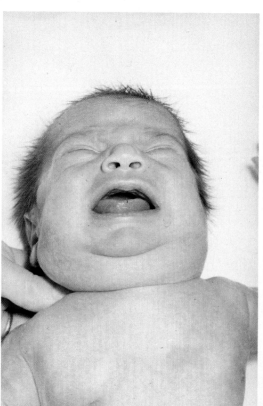

71. Surgical emphysema

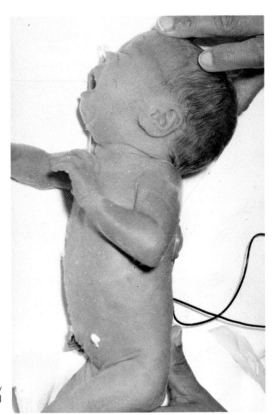

72. Vulnerability of the skin of low birth-weight babies to simple physical insult

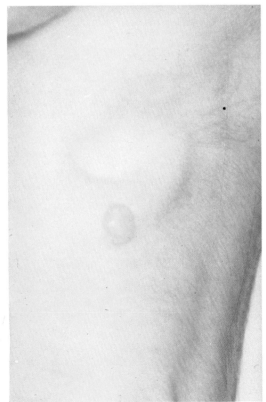

73. Vulnerability of the skin of low birth-weight babies to simple physical insult

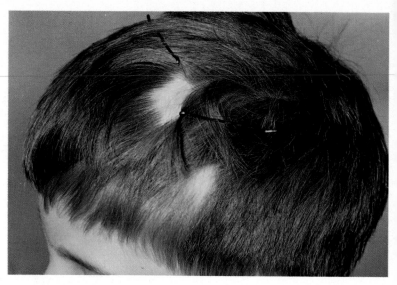

74. Late effects of subdural taps

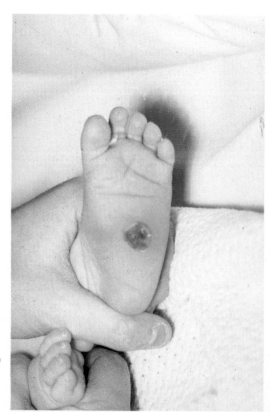

75. Secondary infection of a vaccination
site

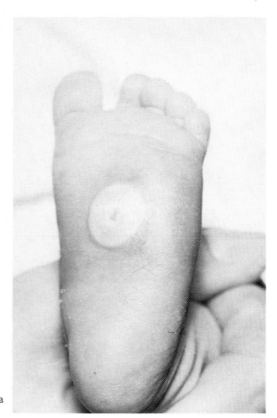

76. Painful inflammatory swelling of a vaccination site

The jittery, restless baby is the one most likely to injure himself by scratching his face (77) or body (78). The risk is greater if he has long nails, which he often has because babies such as he are the very ones likely to be post-term. They can cause abrasions of the cheeks (79), ears (80) or feet (81) by rubbing them against the covers or cot sides. If they are nursed prone, to damp down their hyperactivity, they may in this case rub up abrasions on their noses (82) by head-wagging, or on their knees (83, 84) by repeated hip flexion in a horse-riding movement. Sometimes also, they are inadvertently armed with the instruments of their own downfall in the form of plastic anklets (85) or wristbands. If the baby's face lies in a pool of regurgitated gastric contents, chemical injury can be caused: the neonatal juice is of almost adult strength for a few days after birth and can cause 'vomit burn' (86). Here, too, it is the overactive baby who is most at risk. The burn is often compounded by an abrasion as the baby wriggles in his discomfort (87).

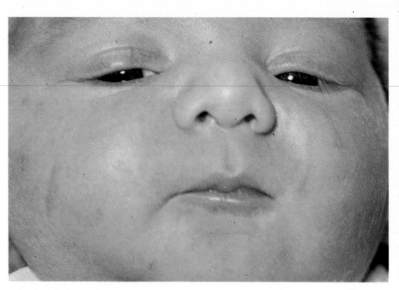

77. Facial scratches self-inflicted by the
restless baby

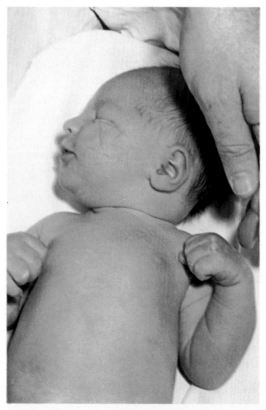

78. Body scratches self-inflicted by the
restless baby

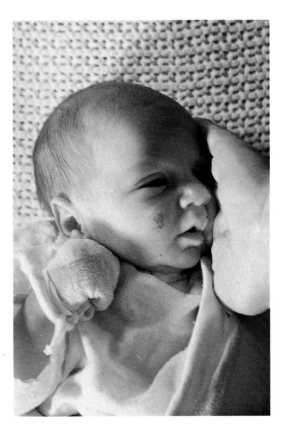

79. Self-inflicted abrasion on the cheek

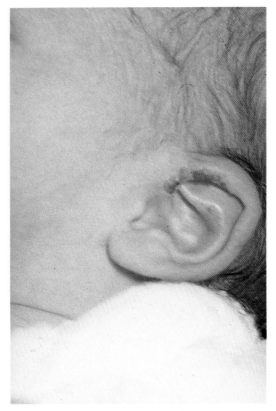

80. Self-inflicted abrasion on the ear

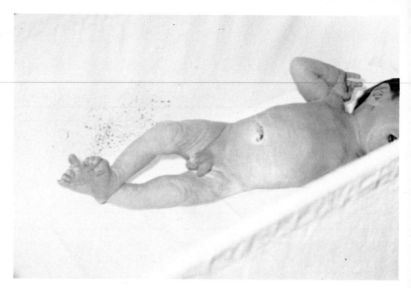

81. Self-inflicted abrasions of the heels

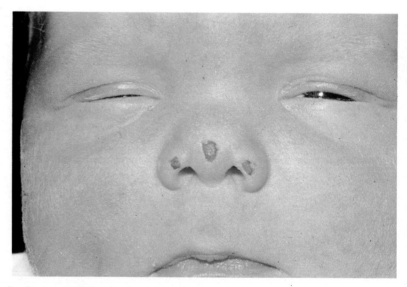

82. Nose abrasions caused by head wagging

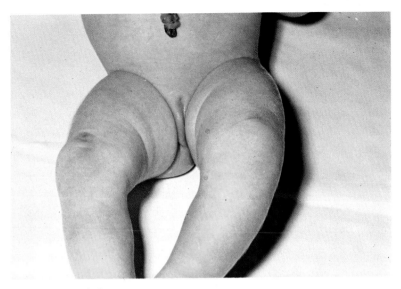

83. Self-inflicted abrasions on the knees

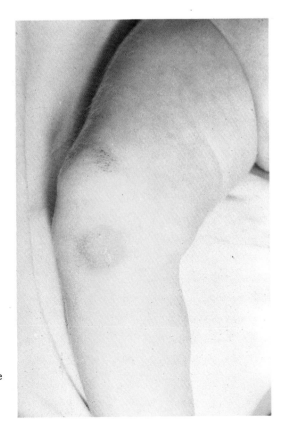

84. Self-inflicted abrasions on the knee

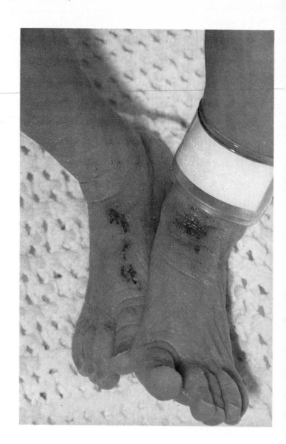

85. Trauma caused by plastic anklet

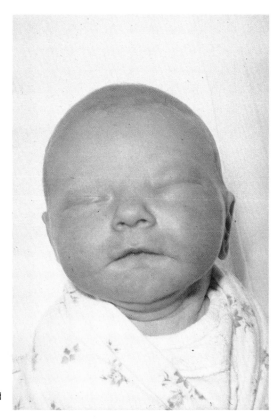

86. Vomit burn from regurgitated
strong neonatal gastric juice

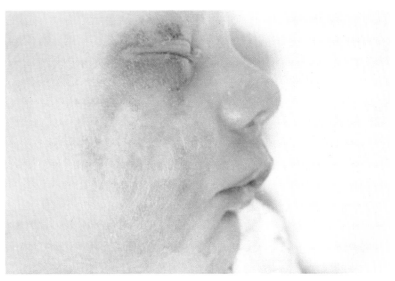

87. Abrasion compounding vomit burn
as the baby wriggles in discomfort

88-90

The commonest trauma is probably transfixion with a safety-pin, another special hazard for the male. Falls, whether straight to the floor or by rolling off a surface (88), can cause bony injuries. Survivors of infanticide attempts also often display traumatic sequelae (89). Damage can be done, too, by the misdirected attentions of young siblings and domestic pets (90: the toddler's welcome home was a karate chop).

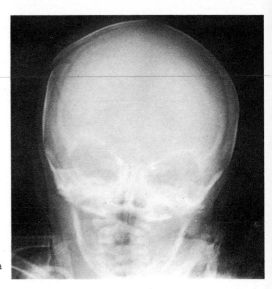

88. Skull injury caused by rolling off a
surface

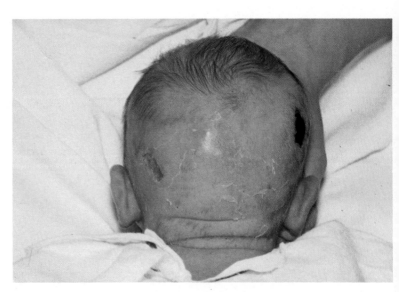

89. Survivor of attempted infanticide

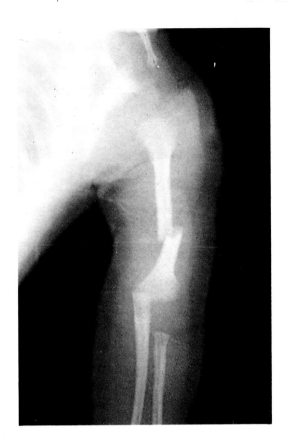

90. Fracture inflicted by sibling

91-93

A 'universal' pattern of Mongolian spot (91) should not be confused with extensive bruising suggestive of the 'battered baby syndrome'. Rarely, a similar birthmark could be misleading in a Caucasian neonate (92); the mother of the baby pictured here had repeated vaginal examinations by medical students to locate the fontanelle. In the event it was several months before they were exculpated (93)! This proved to be the rarity sometimes called the naevus of Ota.

8, 39, 40, 94

If there has been an obstetric procedure, partial thickness congenital skin defects may be thought to be iatrogenic. At birth, however, the rolled edge and fresh granulating base (8) are easily distinguishable from a recent incised wound (39, 40). One mother accused the obstetrician of marking her baby at artificial rupture of the membranes (94). She was confidently assured that the mark was a congenital skin defect, but did not accept the explanation until she saw what the doctor had observed – that there was indeed a much smaller incised wound that the obstetrician *had* caused, lower down on the occiput.

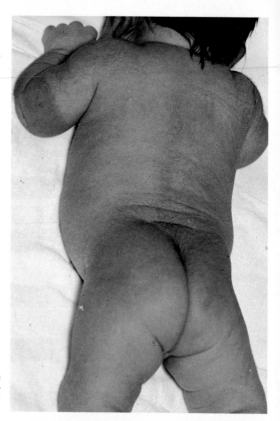

91. A universal pattern of Mongolian spot not to be confused with the extensive bruising suggestive of the 'battered baby syndrome'

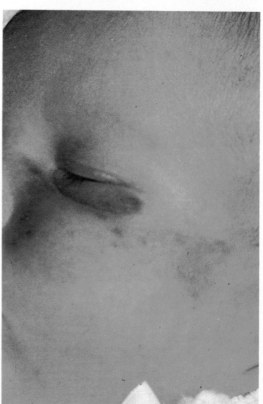

92. A blue birthmark in a Caucasian neonate which could be confused with bruising

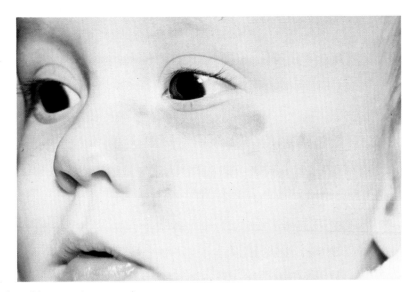

93. Persisting blue marks several months later in the baby shown in plate 92 proved to be the rare naevus of Ota

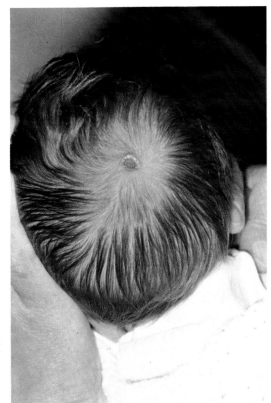

94. Partial thickness congenital skin defect mistakenly thought by the mother to be iatrogenic

Section four

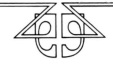

Infection

7

Infectious illnesses in the nursery have declined with the universal observance of barrier nursing principles, especially the obsessional washing of hands with plain soap and water between examinations. Individual infective disorders are a perennial hazard, but even the serious uncomplicated cases usually respond to antibiotics if the diagnosis is not delayed. Unfortunately, the infected baby is often compromised by low birth weight or malformation and the risks may be compounded by the presence of resistant bacterial strains, especially in surgical or intensive care units.

Attention is increasingly directed to prenatal infection, especially in the first trimester when handicap and malformation may be caused. The full range of these infective agents is still being documented and for good management the whole spectrum of clinical and bacteriological expression at and after birth must be defined. In the sixties this was exemplified by the team approach to rubella, which we now expect to prevent by vaccination, and hopefully the same will be possible in the future with other agents such as cytomegalovirus.

The fetus is peculiarly free from infection by common bacteria until shortly before delivery. Instead, he is vulnerable to viruses, protozoa, mycoplasma, fungi or exotic bacteria such as *Listeria*, treponemata, tubercle bacilli, some enteric bacteriae, vibrios or *Brucella*. The outcome, including abortion or stillbirth, will depend mainly upon the maturity of the fetus and the virulence of the infecting agent, the mode of spread of the infection in the mother, the portal of entry into the fetus and his immunological reactivity also affect the situation.

1-4

If fetal infection takes place in the first trimester it can interfere with organogenesis and produce a unique picture of malformation; rubella is the most notorious example, causing defects primarily of eye (1), heart and brain. Throughout pregnancy, the fetus has a reduced capacity for cellular response to infection and the continuing unchecked destructive action of the infecting agent can result in severe pathology (2) unknown in postnatal infection by the same agent. Similarly, infection close to term tends to be more severe (3: chickenpox), although this may not correlate with the mother's condition (4: mild chickenpox, mother was seriously ill with chickenpox pneumonia).

5, 6

When a pregnant woman suffers from an infection potentially harmful to the fetus, one should watch for slowing of the fetal growth rate as a danger signal: an informed examination in the nursery will be oriented in particular to detecting covert signs that might otherwise be overlooked; for example after rubella one would look specifically for retinopathy (5) or osteitis (6).

7-10

The common neonatal warning signs that first alert the clinician may be smallness-for-dates (7: 2360g., 40 weeks estimated gestation), malformations, purpuric (8) or infiltrative (9) rashes, hepatosplenomegaly, jaundice, or unexpected neurological dysfunction perhaps accompanied by microcephaly (10). There may be histopathological evidence of villous placentitis.

11-16

The more ordinary bacterial infections occur shortly before or sometimes during delivery. Congenital purulent meningitis due to *Listeria monocytogenes* apparently spreads by the transplacental route (11). Congenital bacterial pneumonia (12), however, is commonest after prolonged rupture of the membranes, and in this case the infection is more likely to take the cervical-amniotic route. Congenital pustules occur (13-16), and the contents are usually sterile.

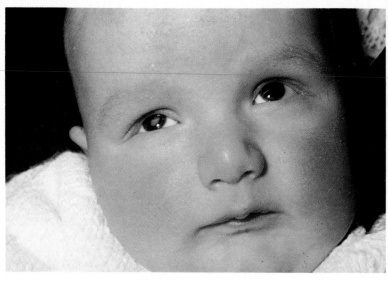

1. Eye defects caused by rubella
infection during the first trimester

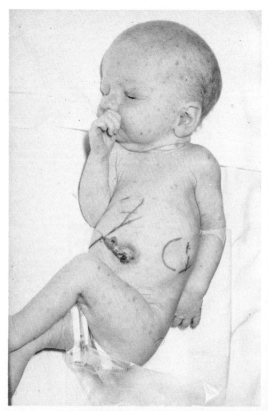

2. Severe pathology following continuing unchecked fetal infection

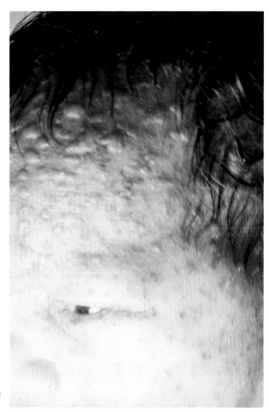

3. Severe chicken pox infection close to term

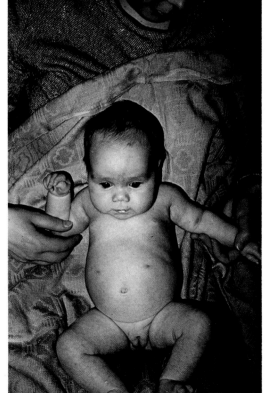

4. Mild chicken pox infection of the infant when the mother was seriously ill with chicken pox and pneumonia

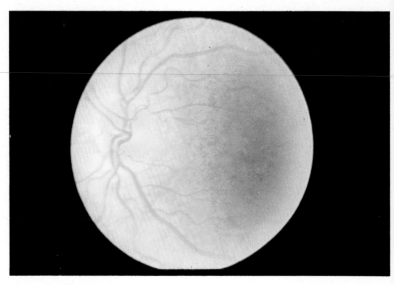

5. Retinopathy following maternal
rubella: 'pepper and salt'

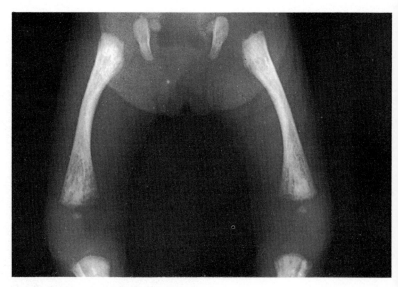

6. Osteitis following maternal rubella:
'celery stalk'

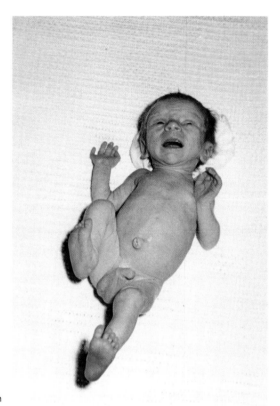

7. Smallness-for-dates associated with prenatal infection

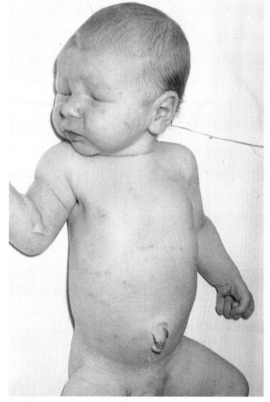

8. Purpuric rash associated with prenatal infection

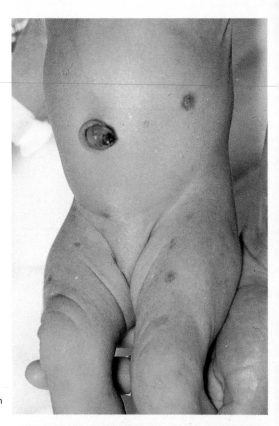

9. Infiltrative rash associated with prenatal infection

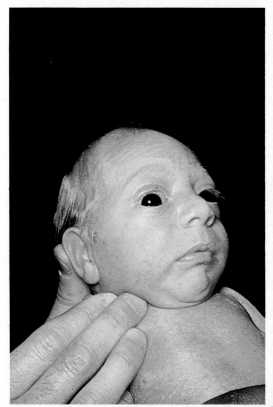

10. Unexpected neurological dysfunction and microcephaly associated with prenatal infection

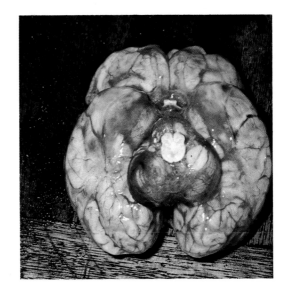

11. Congenital purulent meningitis

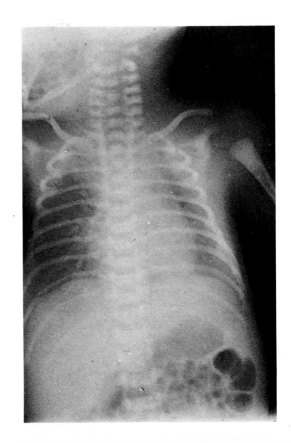

12. Congenital bacterial pneumonia

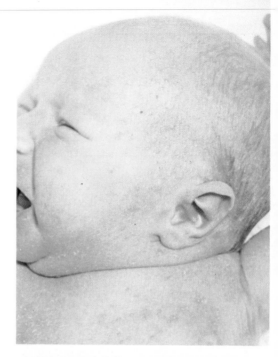

13. Congenital pustules

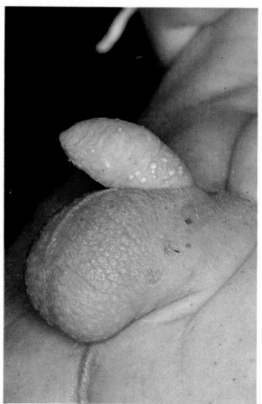

14. Congenital pustules

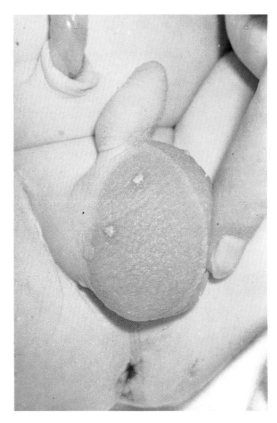

15. Congenital pustules

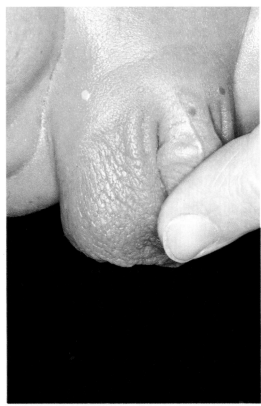

16. Congenital pustules

The intrauterine environment is normally sterile. Within a few days of birth, however, the baby must come to symbiotic terms with the environmental flora, principally staphylococci and *E. coli*. When infection develops these are the organisms most often involved. There is also a special vulnerability to a few other organisms such as *Candida* and *H. influenzae*, or any of the various new 'resident' organisms in our nurseries such as *Pseudomonas* or other opportunists.

Infections like pneumonia or meningitis may present in a fairly 'conventional' way. With other infections, such as those occurring in the urinary tract, a 'conventional' presentation is virtually impossible. The neonate, however, shows unique stereotyped signs of distress; his response to infection may be to develop mottling or peripheral cyanosis, jaundice, oedema or low temperature. The safe rule is that in any case of nonspecific malaise the possibility of infection must be deliberately explored.

The common sites of infection are fairly predictable and can be tabulated in a fashion that parallels the clinical examination:

1. The skin and its appendages
2. The bones
3. The meninges
4. The lungs
5. The urinary tract
6. Anywhere
7. Everywhere

17, 18 The skin and its appendages

In every child the umbilicus is an open site for infection. Mild degrees of cellulitis are acceptable (17) and may facilitate cord shedding. If the condition becomes so severe as to need treatment (18) the possibility of the spread of the infection along the umbilical vein and beyond must be considered.

19-22

If the baby lies in a posture of flexion it is necessary to expose the axillae (19, 20) and groins, because these are moist sites which attract infection. The fingers should be deflexed to look for paronychia (21); the toes (22) are less often affected.

23-25, 70   The eyes are another common site of infection; the
                                       exudative form of superficial conjunctival ophthalmia is
                                       usual (23), it may be gonorrhoeal. There may also be
                                       cellulitis of the loose tissue of the lids (24) or a sty may
                                       form (25). A continuing infection sometimes invades the
                                       lacrimal duct and sets up dacryocystitis (70) in which
                                       there is epiphora and pus issues from the lacrimal
                                       punctum.

26, 27   In the mouth, thrush is the common infection (26). It
                                       forms painful adherent white plaques on the mucosal
                                       surface. It must not be confused with epithelial pearls
                                       or adherent milk (27).

28, 29   Breast hypertrophy can lead to mastitis or abscess
                                       formation (28, 29).

30-35   Skin infection can occur at any site and it is therefore
                                       necessary to inspect the naked baby all over (30, 31).
                                       Cellulitis may develop (32). Sometimes the onset is
                                       multifocal (33) or it may seem to spread more or less
                                       rapidly by inoculation (34, 35).

36-42   The portal for infection may be iatrogenic – medical
                                       help for the baby often tears the skin or epithelium
                                       (36-42).

43   Superficial staphylococcal infection with severe
                                       pustulation and systemic illness is called bullous
                                       impetigo. It should not be confused with the 'scalded
                                       skin syndrome' (43) which is more dangerous; the
                                       debilitated skin rubs off in sheets without pustulation.
                                       This neonatal toxic epidermal necrolysis described by
                                       Ritter is similar to Lyell's disease in later life. It is a
                                       cutaneous response to infection at other sites by
                                       staphylococci of specific phage types.

44-46   The bones   Neonatal osteitis is diagnosed by its two cardinal signs –
                                       inflammatory swelling and pseudoparesis (44). The
                                       response to early treatment is good (45) but cases
                                       treated late have a worse prognosis (46) and relapsing
                                       multifocal infection may result from delays in treatment.

47	The meninges	There may be 'focal' signs such as fits, opisthotonos or a bulging fontanelle to indicate meningitis but unexpected signs of mild but definite neurological trouble (47) may lead to earlier diagnosis, especially when the fontanelle tension is even mildly increased.
48-51		In all cases, especially if an exotic organism is present, the line of closure of the neural tube must be inspected for possible signs of a track; this means careful examination of the midline from the coccyx (48) over the vertex (49, 50) right down to the nasion (51).
52, 53	The lungs	Respiratory difficulty is the best pointer to pneumonia, but quite extensive consolidation (52) may go undetected clinically. Unexplained nonspecific illness requires chest X-ray. (53: bilateral pneumonia, there were no localising clinical signs.)
54	The urinary tract	In cases of infection of the urinary tract, physical examination is unrewarding: a renal swelling (54) or an enlarged bladder may be felt very occasionally and haematuria is exceptional. In cases of jaundice, the urine must be tested for infection.
55-58	Anywhere	The roll-call of uncommon sites for infection is becoming an anatomical catalogue of the parts of the body as widening experience catches the unusual into its net (55, 56). Special circumstances can sometimes cause liability to a particular infection (57: *Pseudomonas* infection, 10th hospital week); occasionally one still finds something that has become a historical curiosity due to improved hygiene (58: gastroenteritis, *E. coli* O 55).
59-67	Everywhere	When several systems or organs are infected more or less simultaneously, septicaemia is common and the baby's survival is in jeopardy (59, 60: urinary tract infection and pneumonia, septicaemia). Most babies can be saved, however, by prompt resuscitative measures and antibiotic treatment. The important thing in the nursery service is to be alert to the early nonspecific signs of malaise (61, 62, 63), especially if the condition deteriorates with minimal handling. When these babies are admitted from outside hospital they are usually seen late and are commonly in extremis (64, 65). If they do survive they are more liable to sequelae (66). The need for haste is paramount: better to have a well and alive baby than a proven case of some catastrophic rarity (67 shows same baby as 64, four months later).

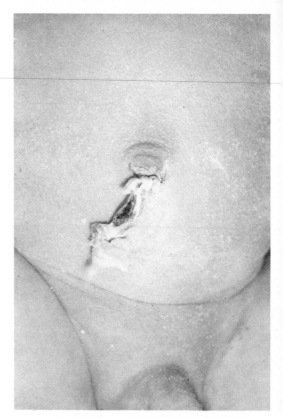

17. Mild cellulitis at the umbilicus

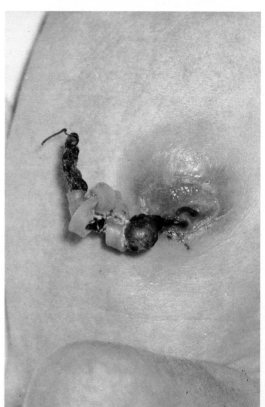

18. Severe cellulitis at the umbilicus

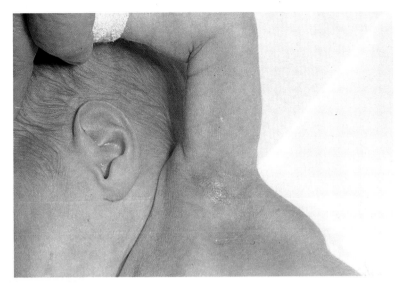

19. Infection of the axilla

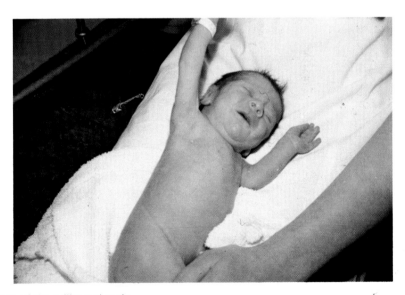

20. Exposure of the axillae and groin
to check for infection in these moist sites

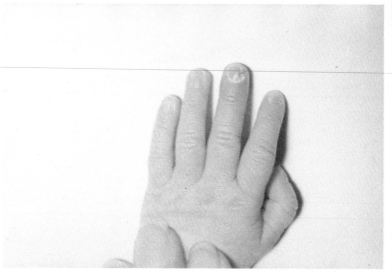

21. Paronychia of the fingers

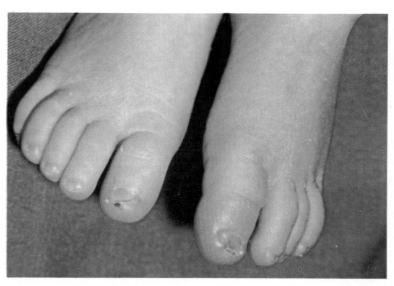

22. Paronychia of the toes

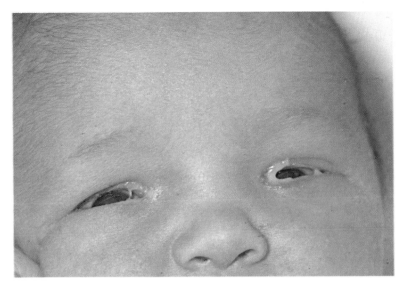

23. Exudative form of superficial conjunctival ophthalmia

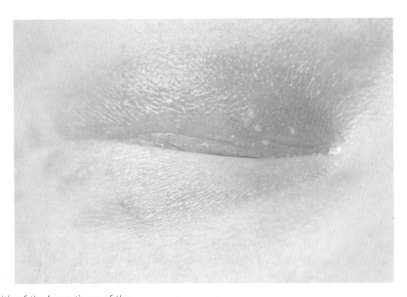

24. Cellulitis of the loose tissue of the lids

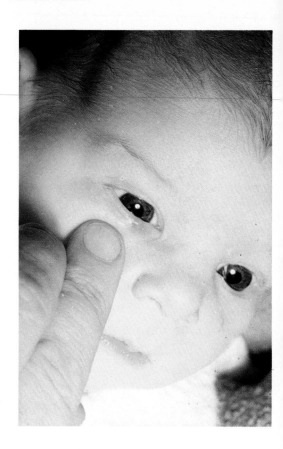

25. Sty

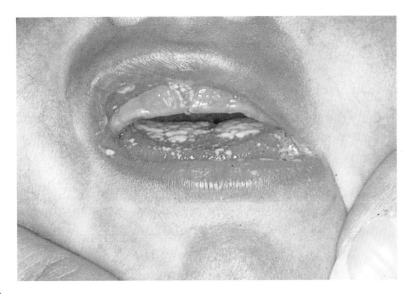

26. Thrush

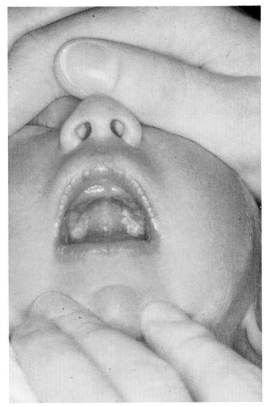

27. Adherent milk and epithelial pearls,
not to be confused with thrush

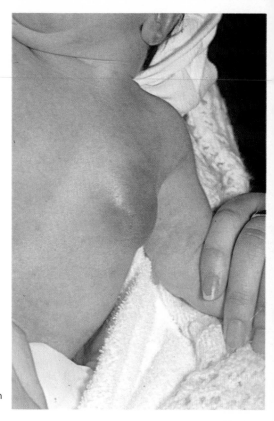

28. Mastitis and abscess formation in breast hypertrophy

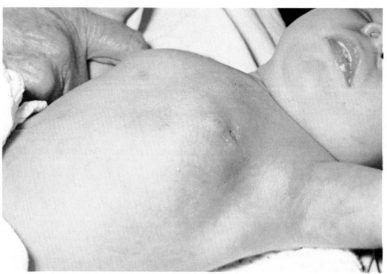

29. After incision

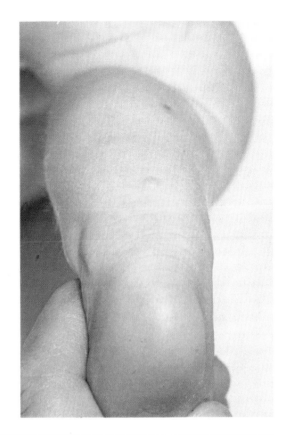

30. Pustule on calf

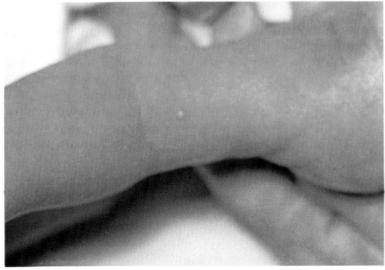

31. Pustule on arm

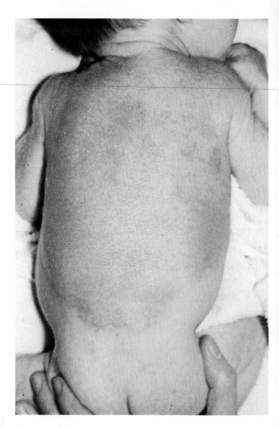

32. Cellulitis over a wide area

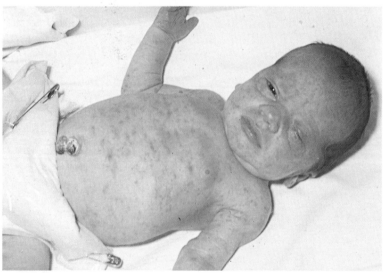

33. Multifocal infection

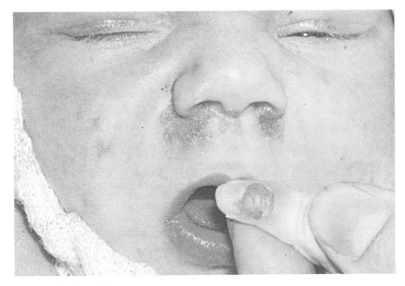

34. Spread of infection by inoculation

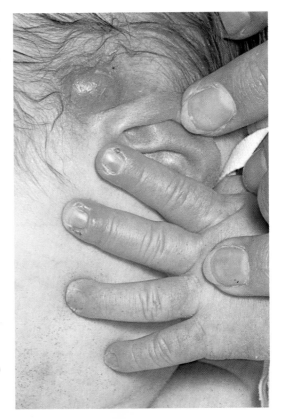

35. Spread of infection by inoculation

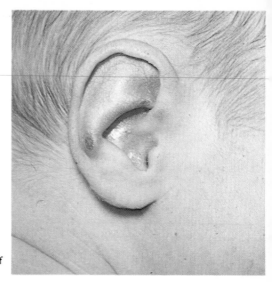

36. Iatrogenic skin tear as a portal of entry for infection of the pinna

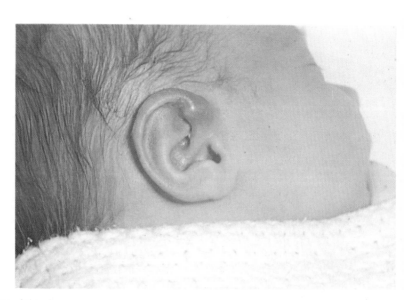

37. Infection of the pinna

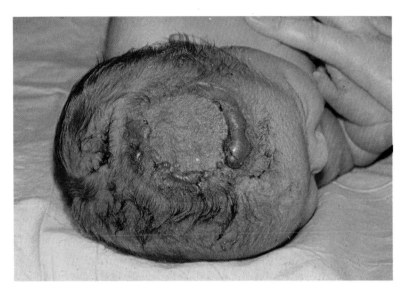

38. Iatrogenic skin tear as a portal of entry for infection of the scalp

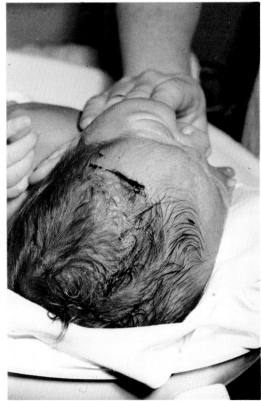

39. Infection of skin tears of the scalp following ventouse extraction

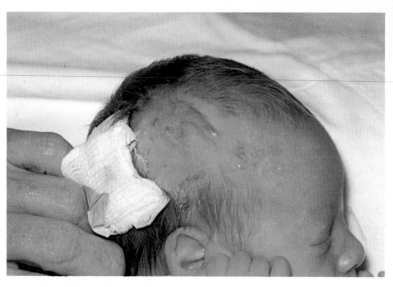

40. Venepuncture sites of the scalp as
portals for infection

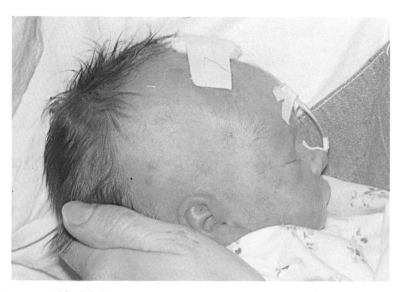

41. Scalp shave as portal for infection

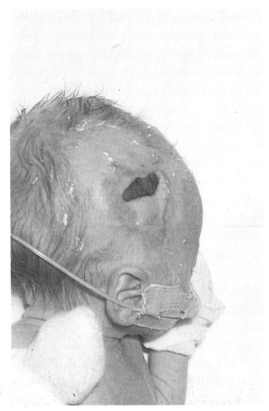

42. Venepuncture sites of the scalp as portals for infection

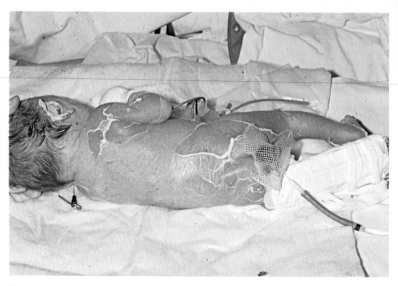

43. 'Scalded skin' syndrome

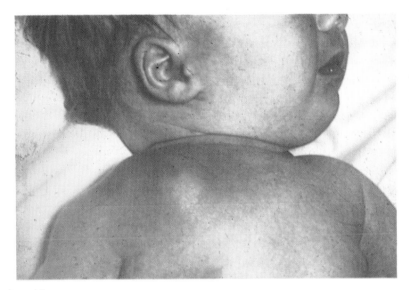

44. Neonatal osteitis

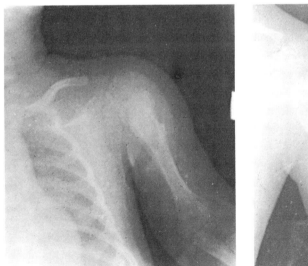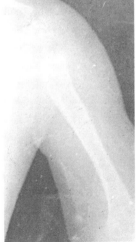

45. Good response of osteitis to early
treatment

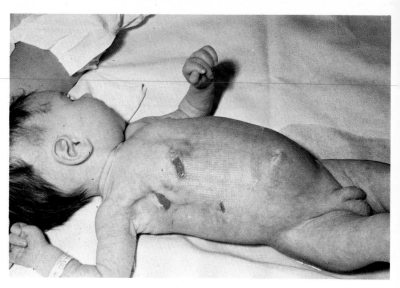

46. Relapsing multifocal infection resulting from delays in treating osteitis

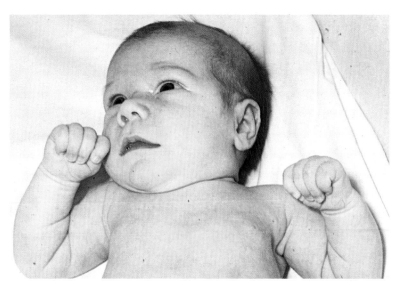

47. Unexpected signs of mild but definite neurological trouble leading to early diagnosis of meningitis

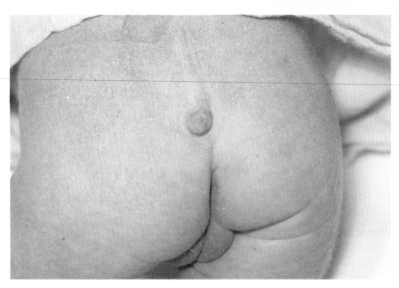

48. Meningitis associated with defects
in the line of closure of the neural tube
in the region over the coccyx

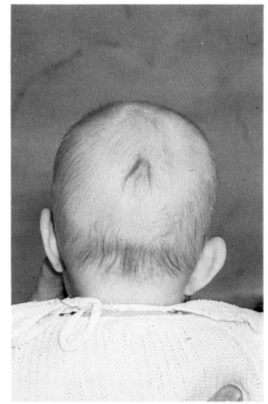

49. Defects in the line of closure of the
neural tube over the vertex

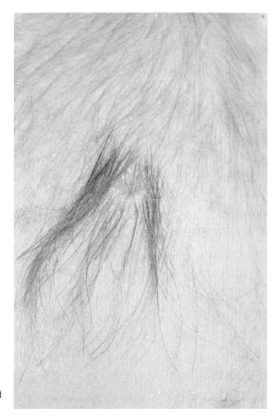

50. Close-up of the defect illustrated in plate 49

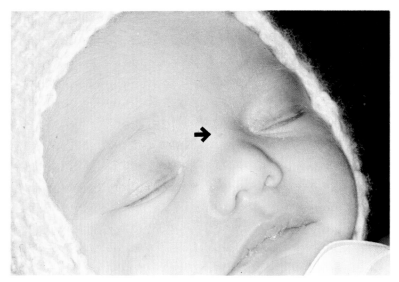

51. Defect in the line of closure of the neural tube at the nasion

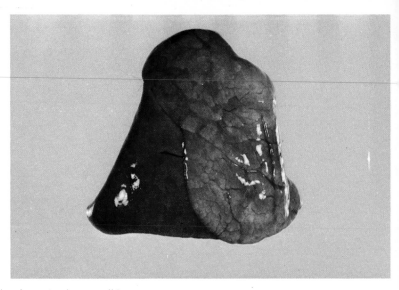

52. Lung showing extensive consolidation from an infant whose pneumonia had gone clinically undetected

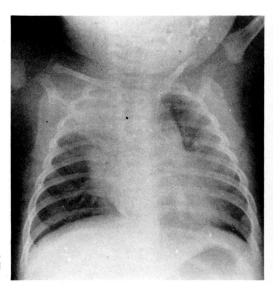

53. Chest X-ray in unexplained non-specific illness revealing bilateral pneumonia

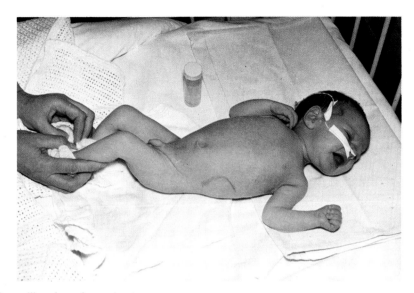

54. Renal swelling in urinary tract
infection

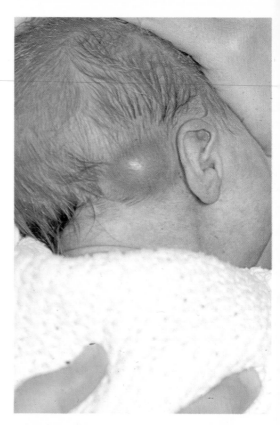

55. Unusual site of infection

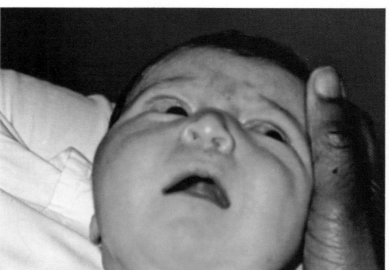

56. Unusual site of infection

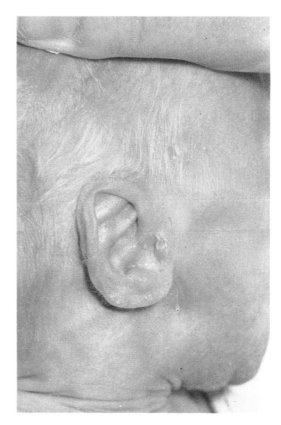

57. *Pseudomonas* infection of the ear

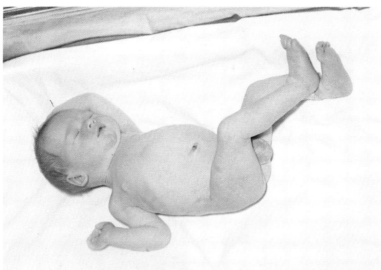

58. Gastroenteritis, *E. coli* O 55

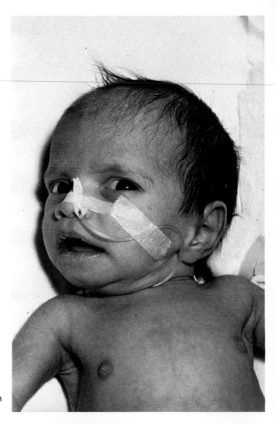

59. Urinary tract infection with septicaemia

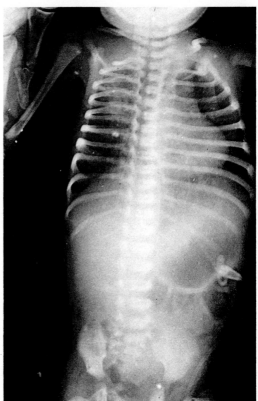

60. Pneumonia with urinary tract infection and septicaemia

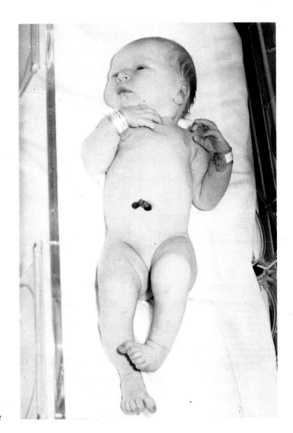

61. Early non-specific signs of malaise

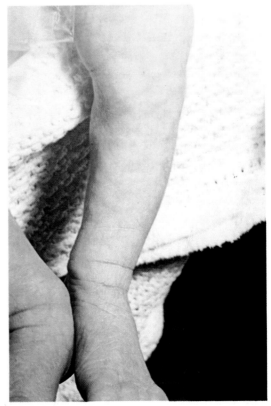

62. Skin mottling

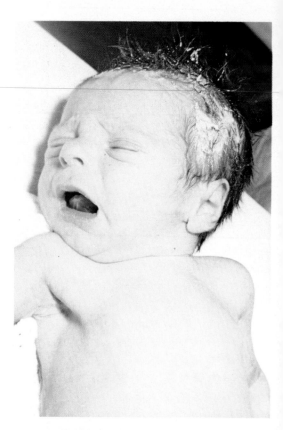

63. Early non-specific signs of malaise

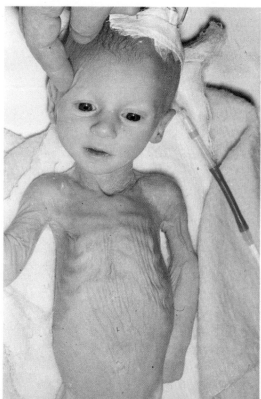

64. Extremely dehydrated baby

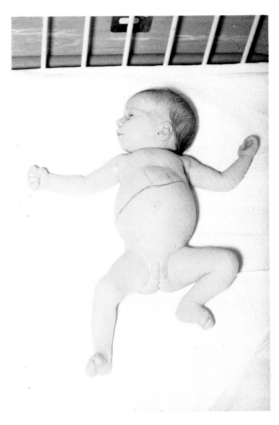

65. Baby in extremis

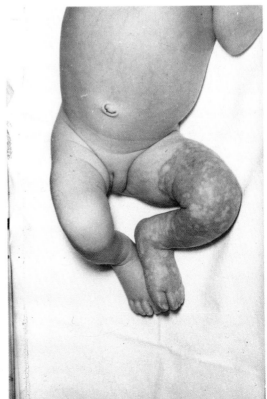

66. Sequel to septicaemia

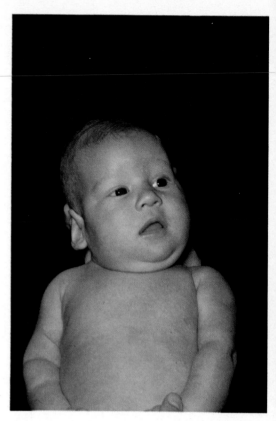

67. The same baby as in plate 64, four
months later

68, 69

Ideally, all survivors of severe prenatal or neonatal infection should be kept under regular review in the early years of life; direct or indirect effects of infection on the nervous system (68) can impair their level of development. A system of 'at risk' registration should be instituted to enable doctors inside and outside hospital to tackle the problem together, particularly in situations where defects like rubella deafness (69) cannot be detected in early infancy.

70, 71

Many late problems, like a discharging eye (70), possible incipient hydrocephalus after meningitis, or asymptomatic relapse of urinary tract infection, are best kept under review in the hospital clinic. For example, pyelography is always needed after neonatal urinary tract infection, since there may be an underlying malformation (71). It should always be borne in mind that neonatal infection may have an inherited cause. This possibility will both influence the management of the child and colour the explanation that the paediatrician will give to the parents about this baby and any they may have in the future.

72, 73

Side-effects of treatment are usually traumatic for the baby because of the risks inherent in investigative and therapeutic procedures. The question of drug toxicity must also be kept in mind. The 'grey syndrome' of chloramphenicol poisoning has become a thing of the past, although one still sees the late dental effects (72, 73: dental staining, U-V fluorescence) of the tetracyclines. Today, this poisoning no longer occurs because other antibiotics are used instead, but the paediatrician must always remain alert to the possibility of early or late toxicity arising from any new drug administered to the newborn.

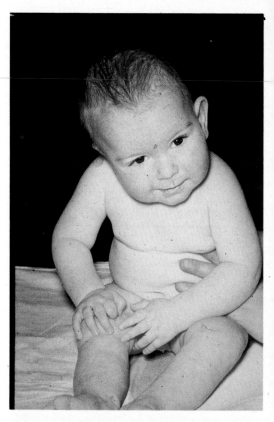

68. Impaired level of development

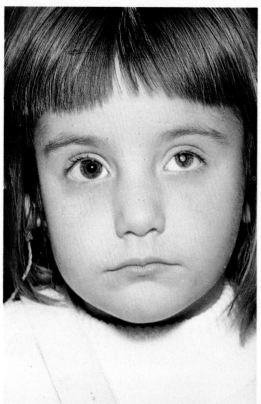

69. Rubella deafness, cataract

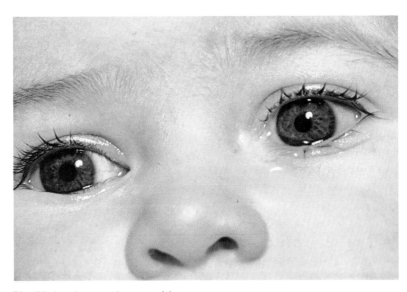

70. Discharging eye, dacryocystitis

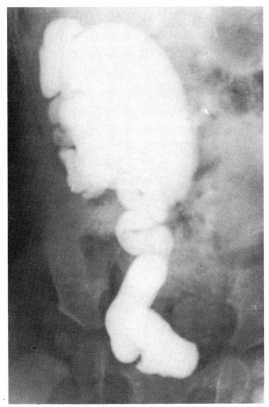

71. Malformation underlying neonatal urinary tract infection

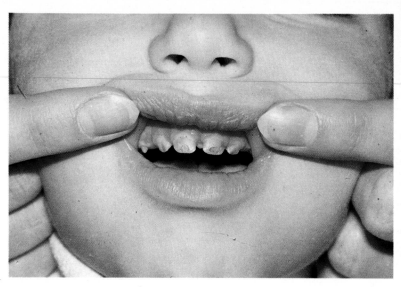

72. Late dental effects of tetracyclines

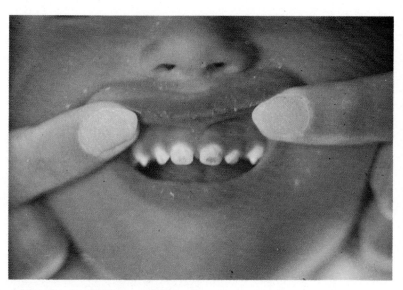

73. Dental staining by tetracyclines
seen with U-V fluorescence

Section five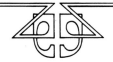

Congenital abnormality

Anomalies of form and structure in the baby at birth are a constant concern of the doctor charged with neonatal care. If the anomalies are severe, they threaten life, and even if the baby survives he may have continuing handicaps or disabilities. The limited success of preventive medicine – universal rubella vaccination, for example, would reduce the total number of severe abnormalities by only 1 per cent – is being offset by the growing number of survivors with spina bifida and other disabilities. A substantial 'hard core' problem appears to be inevitable.

1, 2

The problem is a challenge to all the fundamental paediatric skills. Early diagnosis depends on a sound knowledge of the range of normal. At every stage in management an understanding of the overall situation is essential, and continuing support and advice are often necessary for a whole life-span. Severe abnormality is a serious matter not only for liveborn children and survivors of the perinatal period but must also be taken into account in all cases of stillbirth (Table 1). The survey quoted[1] is far from being the most extensive, but it does have the advantage of practical clinical relevance to the everyday situation in a routine nursery service. Mild abnormality has been briefly dealt with elsewhere in this Atlas among the trivial complaints of the normal newborn baby. Although not in itself serious, it cannot, however, be dismissed; it must be recognised as the possible indicator or harbinger of an associated serious malformation (1, 2: skin tag is the indicator for cleft palate, and hydrocephalus developed soon afterwards).

Abnormality of any degree has four main aspects to be considered:

1. What is the matter?
2. What is the plan?
3. Why did it happen?
4. Could it happen again?

[1]Nelson, M. M., and Forfar, J. O. (1969), 'Congenital Abnormalities at Birth: their Association in the Same Patient' (Develop. Med. Child Neurol., *11*, 3).

Table 1

Major congenital malformations

All deliveries	2.1%
Stillbirth	32.0%
Live births	1.6%
First week deaths	18.0%
Survivors > 1/52	1.3%

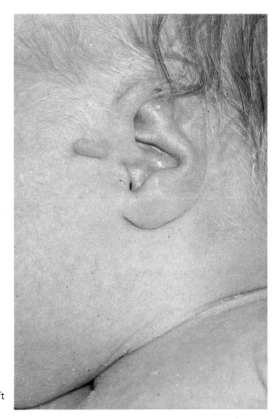

1. Skin tag is the indicator for cleft palate

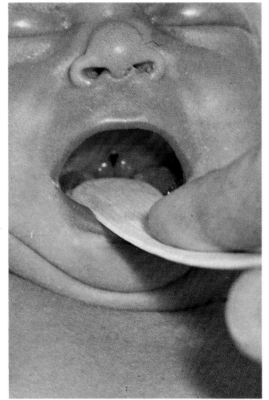

2. Cleft palate in the baby shown in plate 1

3-10

The first question facing the doctor is to define the full physical extent of the immediate problem. With an obvious external presentation, there is no need for expertise at the simple descriptive level, for instance in cases of cleft lip (3), imperforate anus (4), phocomelia (5) or talipes (6). The informed diagnostic search, however, is conducted in the knowledge that malformations are often multiple (Diagrams A, B) especially within a single system or organ (7: atresia of oesophagus and duodenum, dextrocardia and bifid ribs). The presenting abnormality, although potentially lethal, may be correctable, but the same may not be true of the secondary abnormality (8, 9: ventricular septal defect, bilateral hydroureter). Some of the associations between abnormalities are very strong (10: spina bifida, Chiari-Arnold malformation of the hindbrain causing hydrocephalus) and sometimes there is such a predictable grouping that a name can be assigned, as in rubella embryopathy or Down's syndrome.

Diagram A   **Major congenital malformations**

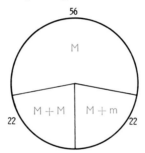

Diagram B   **Minor congenital malformations**

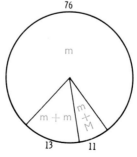

Most abnormalities arise from defects of organogenesis in the first trimester and as such they are true malformations. The doctor's assessment and explanation to the parents involves some knowledge of the fundamental embryological processes, especially of cannulation, midline structure, organ migration and budding or branching.

4, 11-17   Gastro-intestinal tract   Failure of cannulation, with atresia, stenosis or blockage is common. The inherent defects most often affect the oesophagus (11), duodenum and upper small bowel (12) or the terminal large bowel (4). Oesophageal atresia is always suspected in cases of hydramnios, especially when the baby accumulates bubbly mucus in the mouth at birth (11: a plastic tube curls up in the oropharynx and there is excess bubbly mucus in spite of recent aspiration). Bile-stained vomit (13) is a danger signal pointing to obstruction lower down, a 'ladder pattern' of distended loops may be seen through the abdominal wall (14). The mild form of imperforate anus, 'covered anus', can be overlooked if some meconium leaks out on to the perineum (15, 16). A perfectly good lumen may become defective by plication in malrotation, hernia, volvulus or intussusception, it can be blocked in meconium ileus; in Hirschsprung's disease it may be functionally ineffective because of faulty innervation. In this last condition there may not be complete obstruction but if there is a neonatal bowel upset the passage of a meconium plug (17) sometimes provides the vital clue.

18-22   At one stage in pregnancy the midgut migrates into the yolk sac: failure of complete return results in exomphalos; in its severe form it is called omphalocele (18), and hernia into the cord (19) when it is mild. The viscera sometimes protrude through a paraumbilical defect in the abdominal wall – this is called gastroschisis (20) and has a relatively good prognosis. When the gut returns to the abdominal cavity there may be failure of complete normal deployment resulting in 'malrotation', or the viscera may be transposed (21: right-sided stomach, transverse liver). Sometimes the thoracic organs are also involved (22: transverse liver, dextrocardia).

23, 24   Hernia is dangerous if the diaphragm is involved; progressive dilatation of bowel loops in the left chest causes respiratory distress and cyanosis, the lung is collapsed and the mediastinum displaced (23). Occasionally there is a defect in the right side of the diaphragm and the liver herniates, usually through the foramen of Bochdalek (24).

25-27	Genito-urinary tract	Defective cannulation may result in hydronephrosis (25: IVP, bilateral hydronephrosis; 26: cystogram, bilateral reflux defines normal ureters below the pelviureteric junction) or obstruction at the bladder neck or beyond, most often in the male. Anomalous budding and branching is seen in pyelon duplex, which is more common in the female (27: bilateral duplex, massive dilatation of one element on the right, with ureterocele).
28-30		Failure of midline fusion has its extreme expression in bladder exstrophy (28: trigone exposed, complete epispadias with pubic dysraphism). The common mild form is glandular hypospadias with hooded prepuce (29). Inappropriate fusion may occur in the female (30: synechia vulvae which broke down after swabbing).
31-34		Migration may be faulty: the kidney may not ascend (31) or the testicle descend to its proper position (32: undescended testicle; 33: perineal testicle); even the ovary may go astray and end up in the groin (34).
35		A combined disorder arises if the kidneys fuse as they ascend; they may not leave the pelvis or they are sometimes stranded short of their definitive location (35: ectopic fused left kidney overlies L3 vertebra).
36-42, 112		Dysgenesis may affect both kidneys (Potter's syndrome). The extreme form is renal agenesis (36); the facial appearance is characteristic (37), there are limb deformities (38), and even sirenomelia (39). The condition causes oligohydramnios and the fetal surface of the placenta may show amnion nodosum (40). The fatal lesion is pulmonary hypoplasia (112). The condition is usually sporadic but occasionally recessively determined (41, sibling of no. 38). A complete unilateral defect is not in itself serious (42: the baby succumbed to associated abnormalities) and hypoplasia with normal miniature architecture goes undetected for years.
43-46		Anomalous genitalia may be more or less neutral in either sex (43: cloaca with rudimentary phallus in a girl). There is a wide spectrum of distortion in both the female (44, 45: virilisation in the common form of adrenal hyperplasia) and the male (46: feminisation in the very uncommon form of lipoid adrenal hyperplasia).

47-55	Nervous system	The neural tube closes by infolding along the midline from the coccyx to the nasion, and defects of fusion can occur anywhere along this line. The lumbar region is the commonest site (47). Due regard, therefore, must be paid to any trivial abnormalities along this line of closure, as they could be the tip of an iceberg (48-54): naevi, sinuses, lumps and hairtufts are dangerous (55: a cord running from a dermal sinus into the vertebral canal, associated with a lipoma).
56, 130		Deficient neuronal development in the brain due to heredity, infection or irradiation may result in microcephaly. This may be obvious (130) or can appear in a less evident form (56) which would only be revealed for the less experienced doctor by routine head circumference measurement in the nursery.
57-60		Extensive developmental defects in the higher parts of the brain may have an open cranium (57: anencephaly) or a closed cranium (58: hydranencephaly). The doctor will suspect the latter condition if severe unexplained neurological dysfunction is discovered: the skull should be transilluminated to look for the 'Chinese lantern' sign (59, 60).
61		Disordered cannulation may involve the Sylvian aqueduct or fourth ventricle exit foramina, with resulting hydrocephalus (61).
62-74	Skeletal	Defective budding and branching affecting limb development may extend proximally (62) or to an intermediate level (63), or may be confined to the periphery (64). Amniotic bands or tears (65) can theoretically play a part in causing some of these segmental defects and amputations. Digital differentiation may be anomalous: oligodactyly (66, 67), or polydactyly (68) or varying degrees of syndactyly (69-74).
75-78, 89		Intrauterine compression often causes skeletal abnormalities of mild degree; the common serious problem is talipes requiring orthopaedic treatment (75). 'Bent bones' usually have an associated dimple which has grown away from the angle by the time of delivery (76). Severe compressional disorders usually

stem from some bizarre intrauterine situation (77). Sometimes one is not sure what role is played by external pressure (78: arthrogryposis; 89: Pierre Robin syndrome of retrognathos with cleft palate; the tongue is floppy and may suffocate the baby).

79-82 Generalised disease of the skeleton may present with short (79: achondroplasia) or deformed (80: osteogenesis imperfecta) limbs and the facial appearance may be unusual (81: 'gargoylism', generalised gangliosidosis). Prenatal radiological diagnosis is possible in many instances (82: osteogenesis imperfecta; only the base of the skull is visualised at term).

83 Abnormality of the skull is serious because there is often synostosis, a usually conspicuous cosmetic disorder, and vision may be affected (83: Crouzon's disease).

3, 84-96 The face The normal anatomy is formed by the union of branchial arch processes which grow in from the sides to fuse in the middle and the common local anomalies are defects of midline structure. The lip or palate may be affected on one or both sides (84, 85, 3) or in the midline (86) and combined lesions often occur (87, 88). They could be caused by a defect of the Stapedial artery, which supplies the first branchial arch, and these clefts, together with some related abnormalities, are sometimes grouped together as 'first arch syndromes'. The Pierre Robin syndrome (89) is one. Mandibulofacial dysostosis together with malformation of the external ears (90, 91) is common to a small group of which the Treacher-Collins syndrome is best known, it includes an antimongoloid slant to the eyes (92), clefts in the lower lids and pits in the cheek (93). Waardenburg's syndrome shows a white forelock (94) with heterochromia iris and dystopia canthorum (95) and the eyebrows meet in the midline (96). These are not just interesting curiosities: Waardenburg carries a 1-in-3 risk of deafness, Treacher-Collins deafness can be partly alleviated by reconstructive surgery, and the Pierre Robin syndrome involves an intrinsic risk of mental slowness.

97-108   Chromosomal   The commonest of these conditions have highly
                abnormalities   characteristic external appearances. Down's trisomy-21
                                     is the best known (97). Patau's trisomy-13 presents
                                     severe harelip, cleft palate with eye defects (98),
                                     polydactyly (99), partial thickness scalp defects (100)
                                     and single umbilical artery (101). Edwards's trisomy-18
                                     is recognised by micrognathos and low-set ears (102,
                                     103), 'rocker bottom' feet (104) and fingers held in
                                     a typical overlapping posture (105). Turner's (XO)
                                     syndrome is easy to recognise in a florid form if there is
                                     neck webbing with a 'trident' hairline (106, 107); most
                                     cases are inconspicuous in the nursery but this
                                     syndrome should always be suspected in females with
                                     congenital lymphoedema and hypoplastic
                                     toenails (108).

109   The main neonatal risk in Down's syndrome is from
                                     congenital heart disease (109) and duodenal atresia.

110   Dermatoglyphic disorders are common and may help
                                     diagnosis in doubtful cases; the best known is distal
                                     migration of the proximal triradial point in Down's
                                     syndrome. A universal 'low arch' fingerprint pattern
                                     (110) is characteristic of Edwards's syndrome.

111   Cardiovascular   Abnormalities are common – occurring in up to 7 per
                system   1000 live births; they epitomise the whole problem
                                     of congenital abnormality in their embryological
                                     mechanisms, multiplicity within the organ or system
                                     and frequent association with malformation elsewhere.
                                     They are usually found during routine examination
                                     and must be suspected in any nonspecific form of
                                     nursery illness from slow feeding to going dusky on
                                     vigorous crying (111).

112   The lungs   Isolated pulmonary abnormality is rarely diagnosed
                                     in the nursery unless serious illness develops from
                                     uncommon disorders such as obstructive lobar
                                     emphysema or a tension cyst. The common disorders
                                     are associated with other abnormalities, such as
                                     hypoplasia due to a severe defect of budding (112:
                                     in Potter's syndrome, this is the lethal defect, the
                                     child not surviving long enough to develop uraemia).

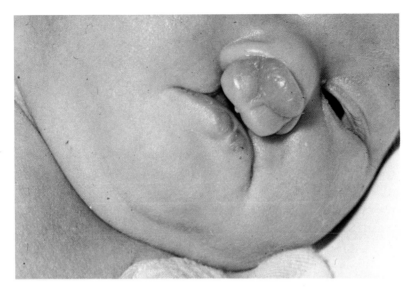

3. Cleft lip

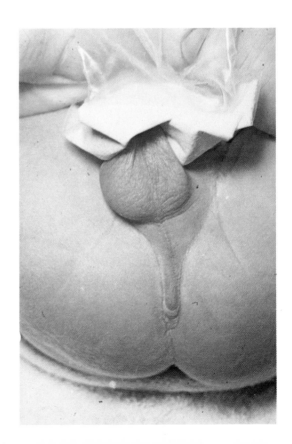

4. Imperforate anus

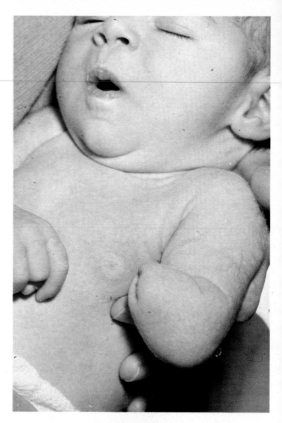

5. Phocomelia

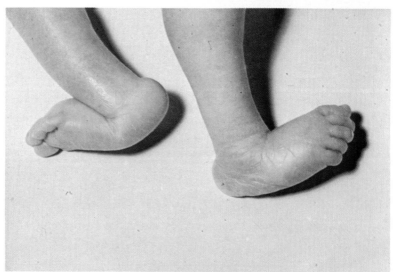

6. Talipes

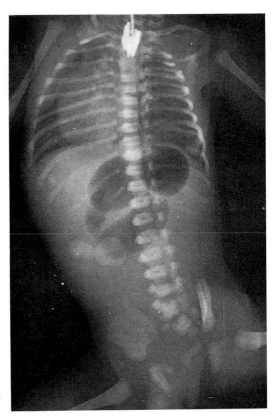

7. Atresia of oesophagus and duodenum, dextrocardia and bifid ribs

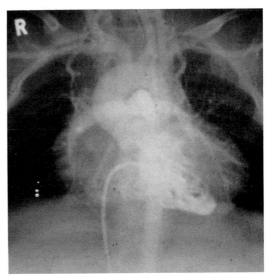

8. Presenting abnormality of ventricular septal defect

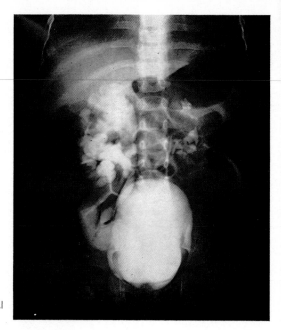

9. Secondary abnormality of bilateral hydroureter

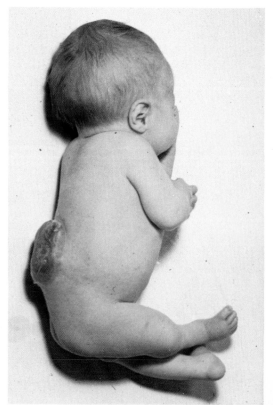

10. Spina bifida with Chiari-Arnold malformation of the hindbrain causing hydrocephalus

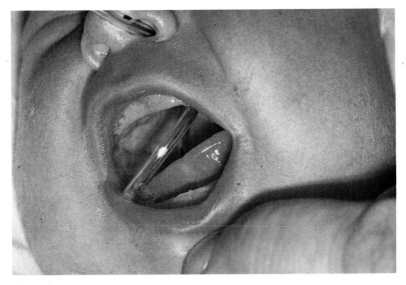

11. Oesophageal atresia

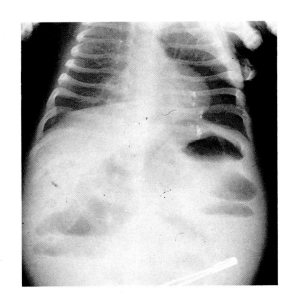

12. Upper small bowel obstruction

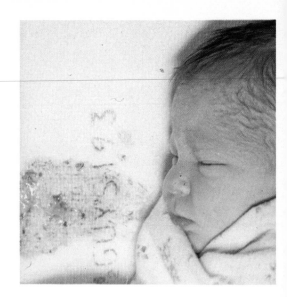

13. Bile stained vomit

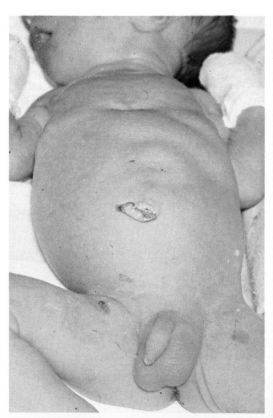

14. 'Ladder pattern' of distended
loops of bowel seen through the
abdominal wall

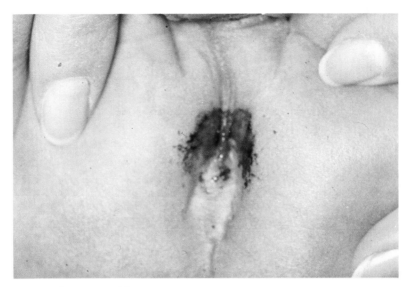

15. Mild form of imperforate anus with leaking meconium

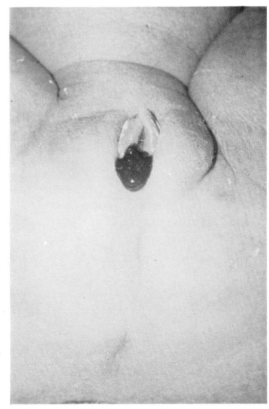

16. Imperforate anus with meconium leaking from vagina

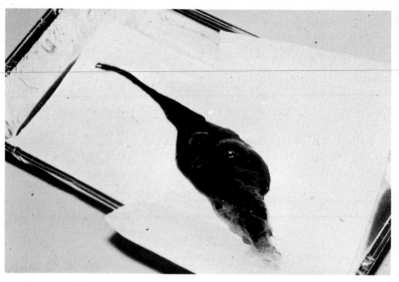

17. Meconium plug passed during a neonatal bowel upset is a clue to Hirschsprung's disease

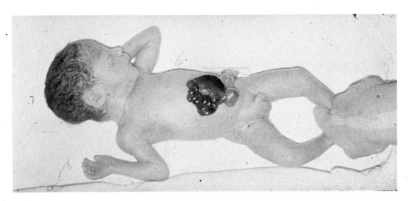

18. Omphalocœle

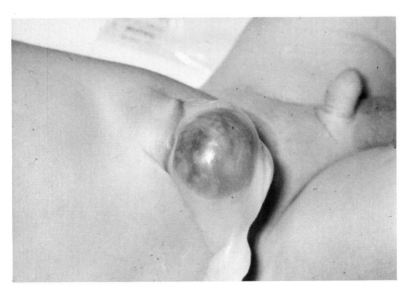

19. Hernia into the cord

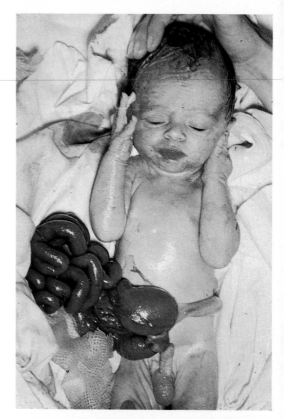

20. Gastroschisis

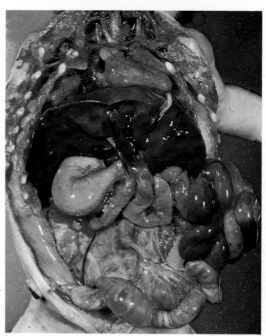

21. Transposed viscera: right-sided
stomach, transverse liver

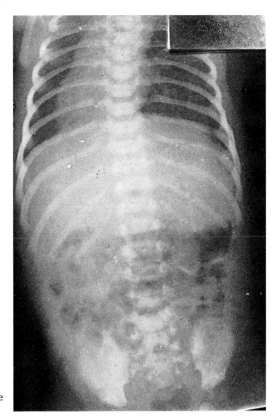

22. Transposed viscera: transverse
liver with dextrocardia

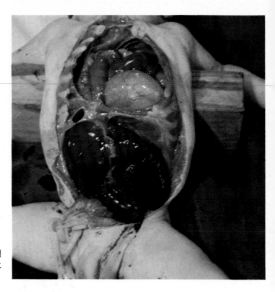

23. Collapsed lung and displaced mediastrinum due to diaphragmatic hernia

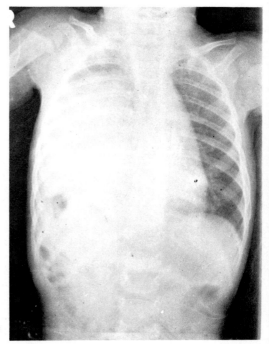

24. Hernia of the liver into the thoracic cavity

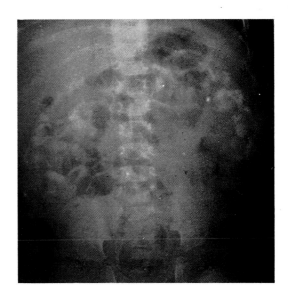

25. IVP, bilateral hydronephrosis

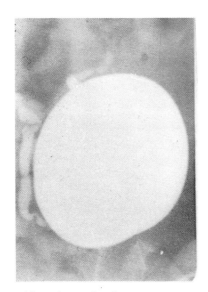
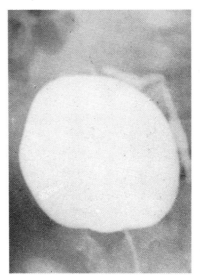

26. Cystogram, bilateral ureteric reflux

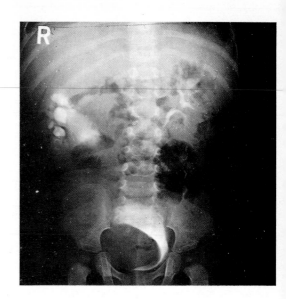

27. Pyelon duplex, ureterocele

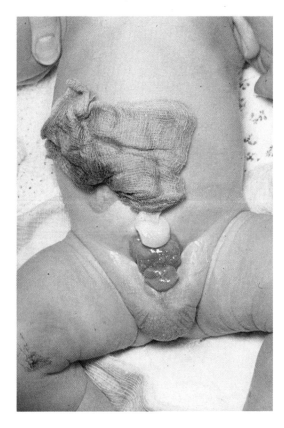

28. Bladder extrophy

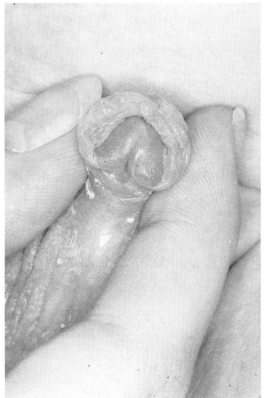

29. Glandular hypospadias with hooded foreskin

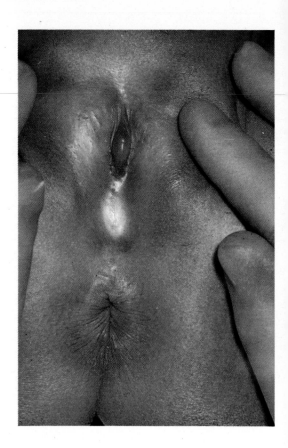

30. Synechia vulvae

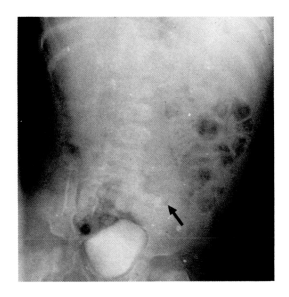

31. Unascended kidney

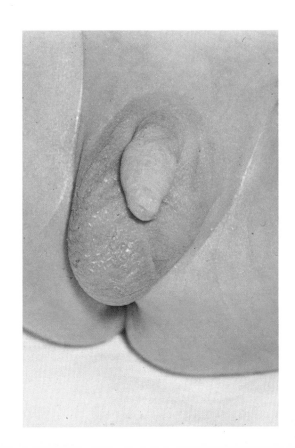

32. Undescended testicle

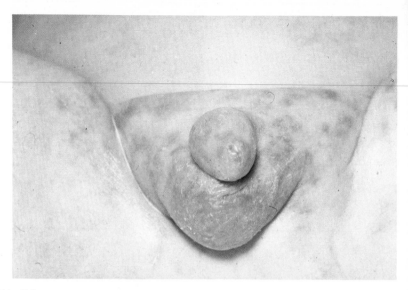

33. Perineal testicle

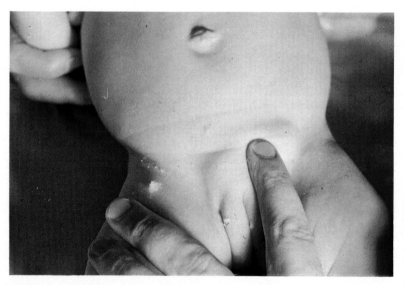

34. Ovary misplaced in the groin

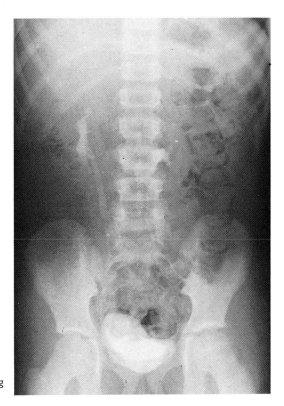

35. Ectopic fused left kidney overlying
L3 vertebra

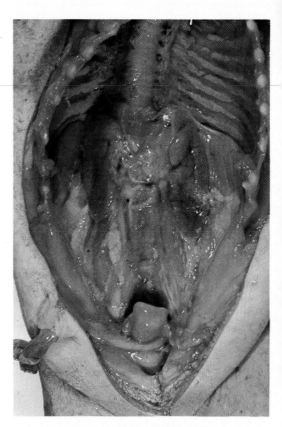

36. Renal agenesis in Potter's syndrome

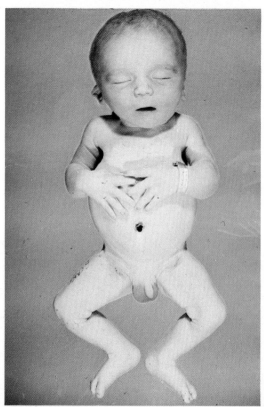

37. Characteristic facial appearance in
Potter's syndrome

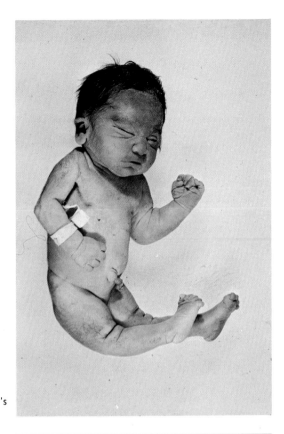

38. Limb deformity in Potter's syndrome

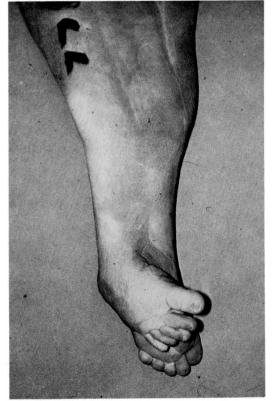

39. Sirenomelia in Potter's syndrome

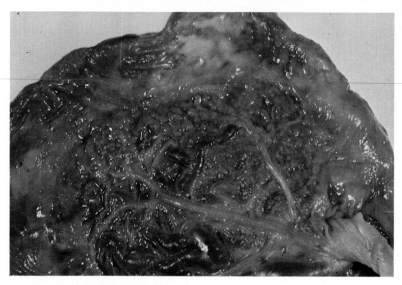

40. *Amnion nodosum* on the fetal surface
of the placenta in Potter's syndrome

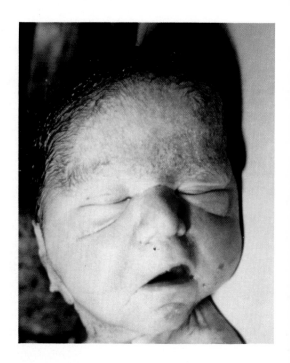

41. Sibling of the baby in plate 38

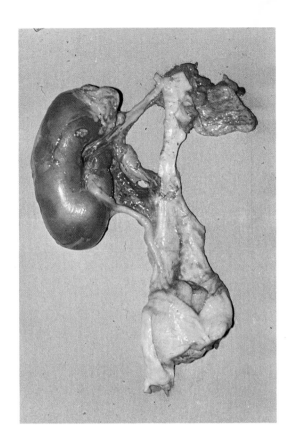

42. Unilateral renal agenesis

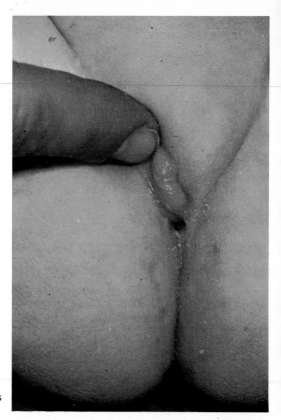

43. Cloaca with rudimentally phallus
in a girl

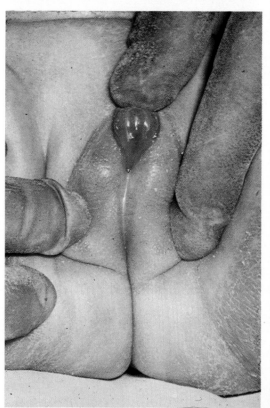

44. Virilisation in adrenal hyperplasia

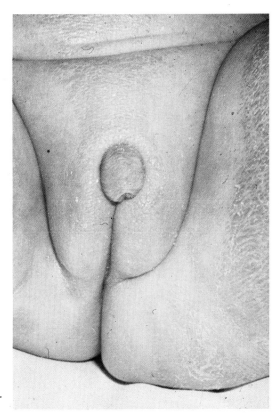

45. Virilisation with adrenal hyperplasia

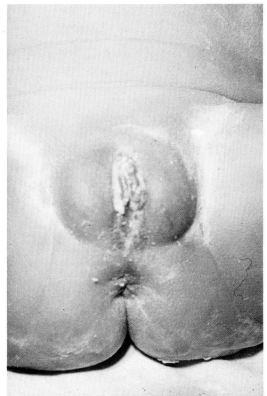

46. Feminisation in lipoid adrenal
hyperplasia

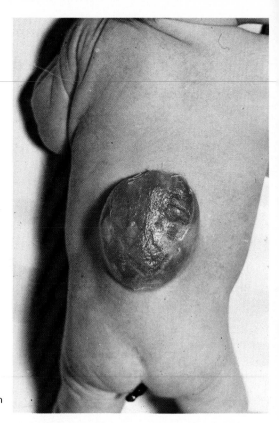

47. Defect of neural tube closure in
the lumbar region

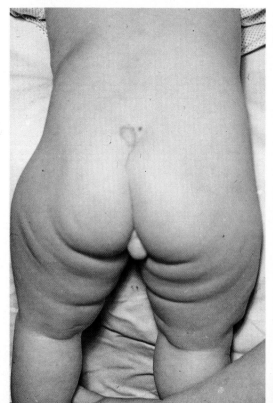

48. Naevus in the midline of the lumbar
region

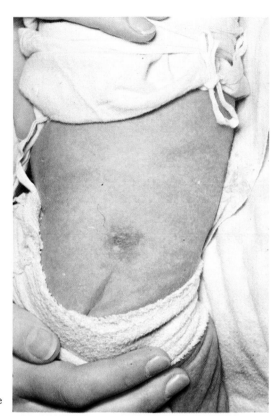

49. Skin defect in the midline of the lumbar region

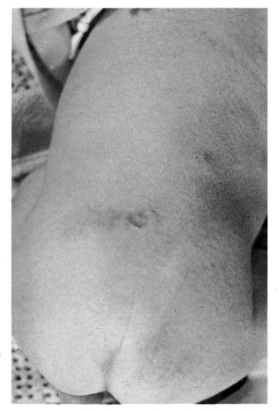

50. Skin defect in the midline of the lumbar region

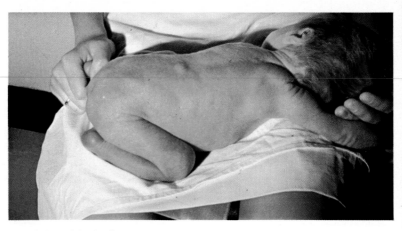

51. Lump in the midline of the lumbar
region

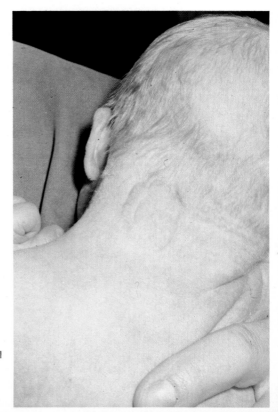

52. Lump in the midline of the cervical
region

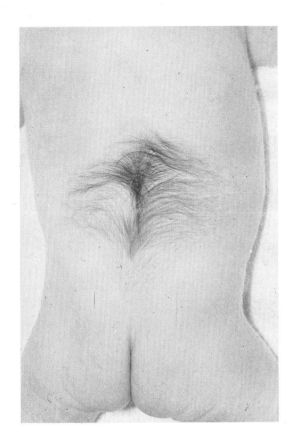

53. Hair tuft in the lumbar region

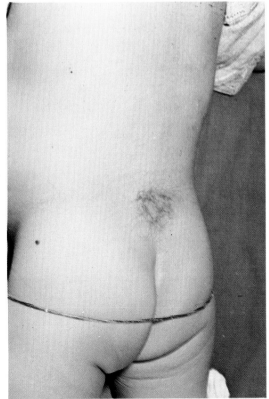

54. Hair tuft in the lumbar region

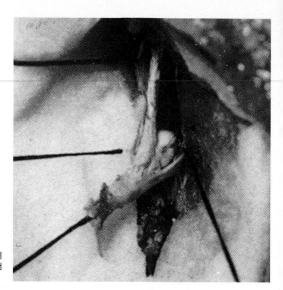

55. A cord running from a dermal sinus into the vertebral canal, associated with a lipoma

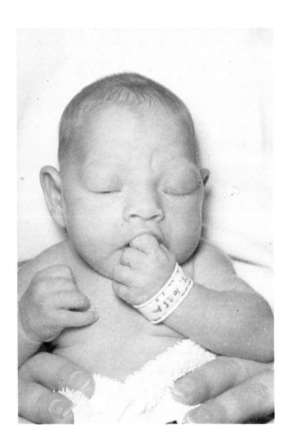

56. Microcephaly of mild degree

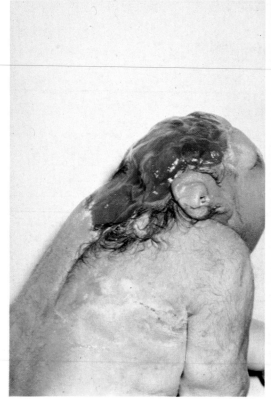

57. Anencephaly

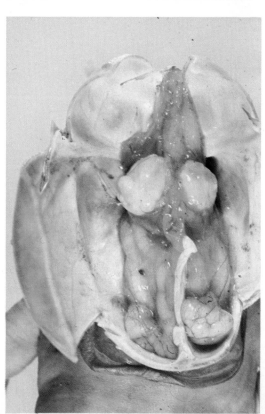

58. Hydranencephaly

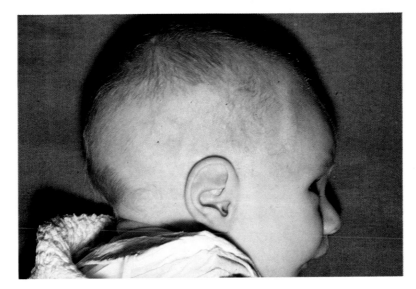

59. Hydranencephaly

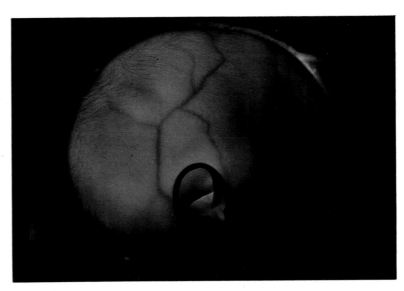

60. 'Chinese   lantern'   sign   of
hydranencephaly

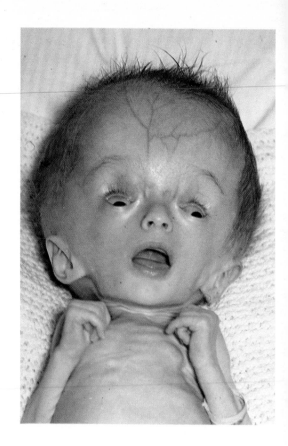

61. Hydrocephalus

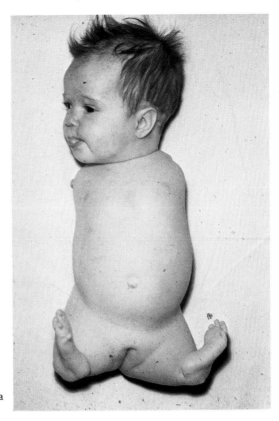

62. Amelia of the arms and phocomelia of the legs

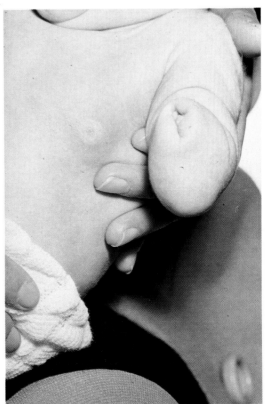

63. Phocomelia of one arm

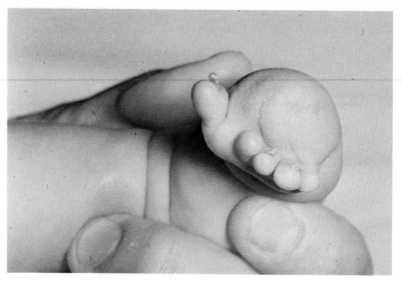

64. Peripheral defect in limb development

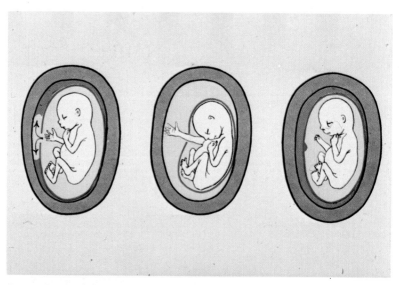

65. Amniotic tear

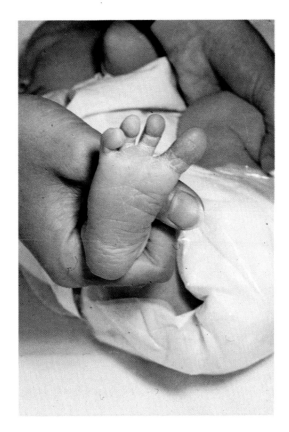

66. Oligodactyly

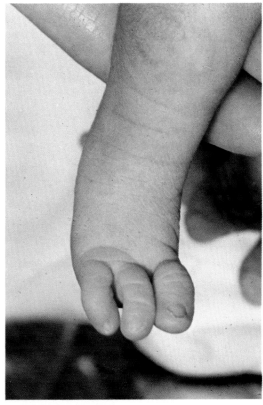

67. Oligodactyly

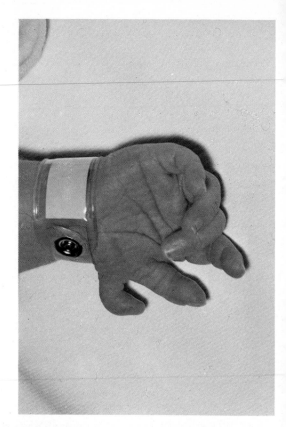

68. Polydactyly

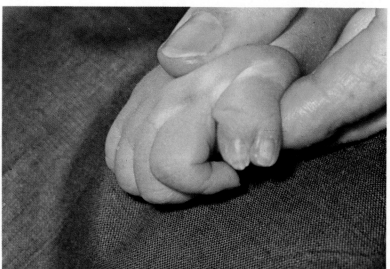

69. Polydactyly/syndactyly

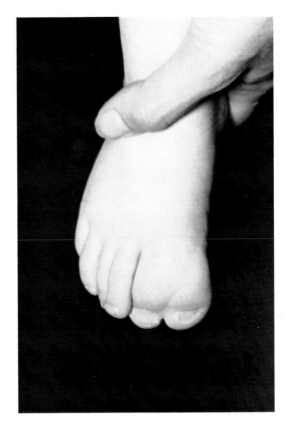

70. Polydactyly/syndactyly

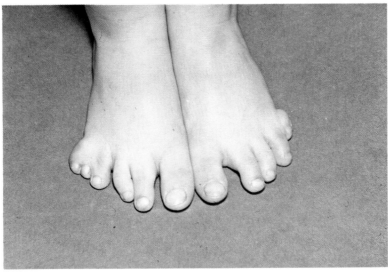

71. Polydactyly/syndactyly

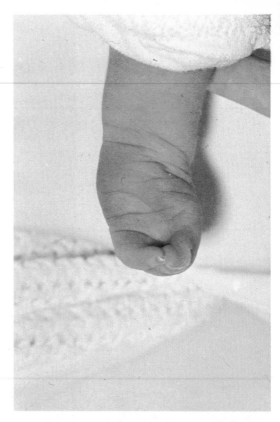

72. Syndactyly

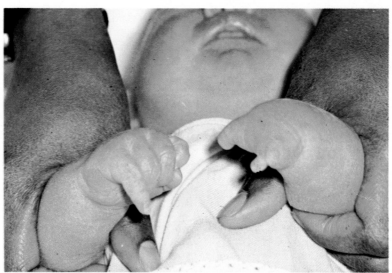

73. Syndactyly

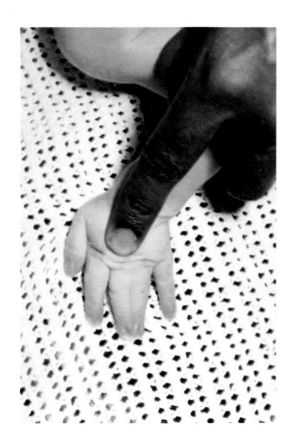

74. Syndactyly

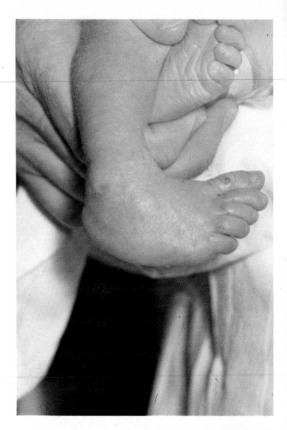

75. Talipes

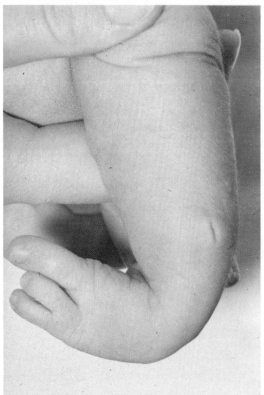

76. Dimple associated with 'bent bones'; oligodactyly

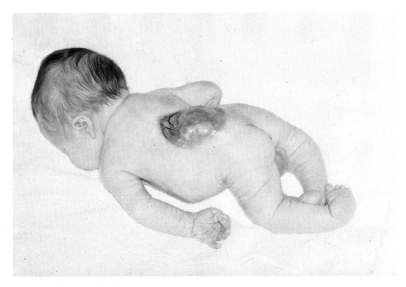

77. Severe compressional disorder
with myelomeningocele

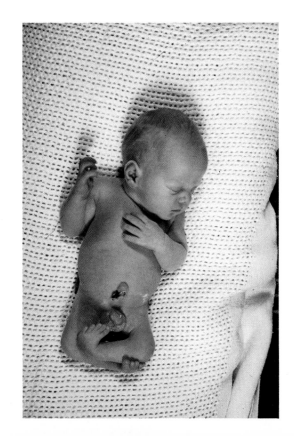

78. Arthrogryposis

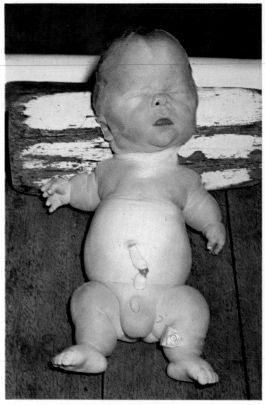

79. Achondroplasia

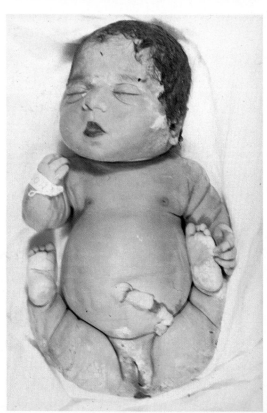

80. Osteogenesis imperfecta

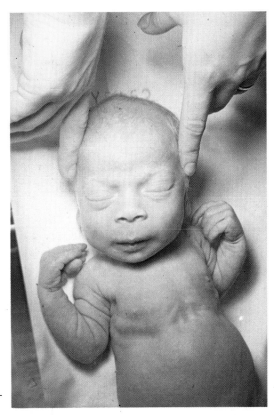

81. Gargoylism, generalised ganglio-sidosis

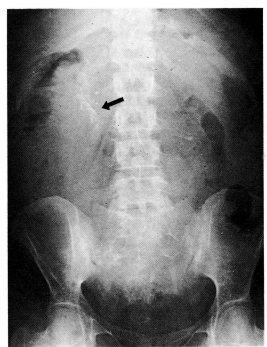

82. Prenatal roentgenogram showing osteogenesis imperfecta. Base of skull arrowed

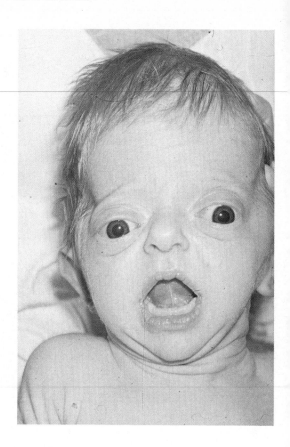

83. Crouzon's disease

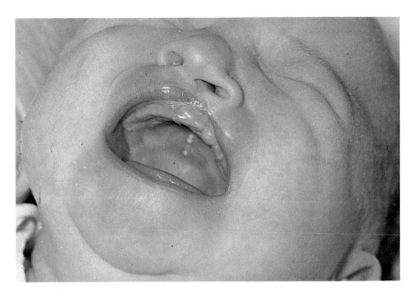

84. Cleft lip

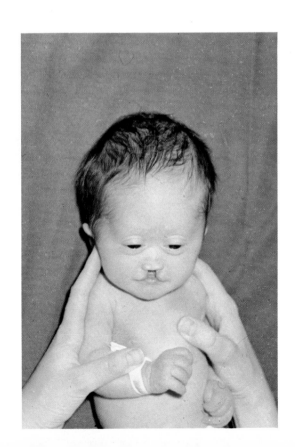

85. Cleft lip

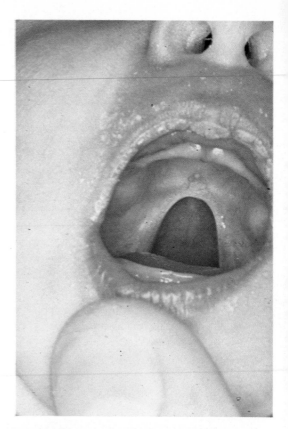

86. Cleft palate

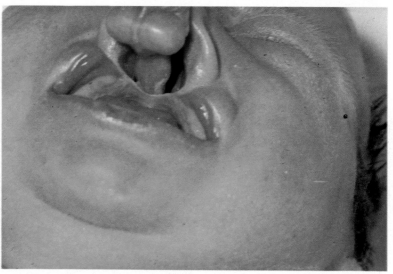

87. Combined cleft lip and cleft palate

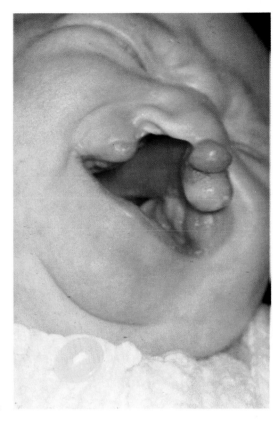

88. Combined cleft lip and cleft palate

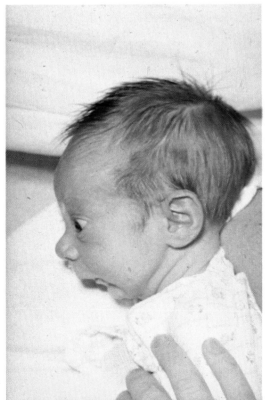

89. Pierre Robin syndrome

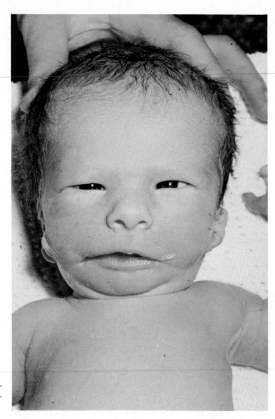

90, 91. Mandibulofacial dysostosis, malformation of the external ears, Treacher-
Collins syndrome

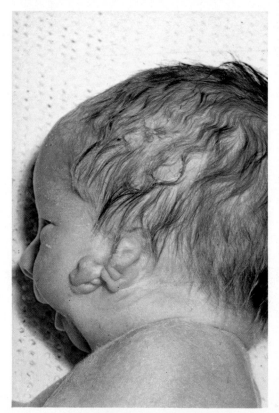

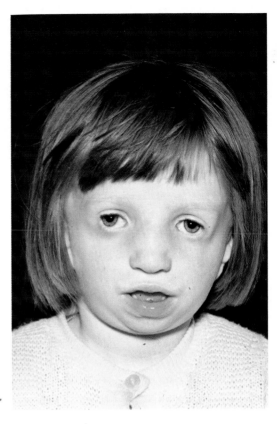

92. Antimongoloid slant to the eyes, Treacher-Collins syndrome

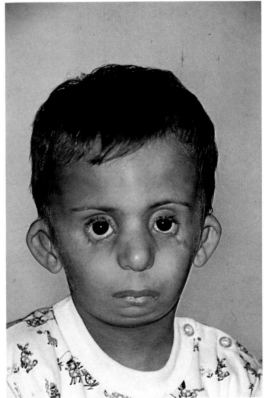

93. Clefts in the lower lids and pits in the cheeks, mandibulofacial dysostosis, Treacher-Collins syndrome

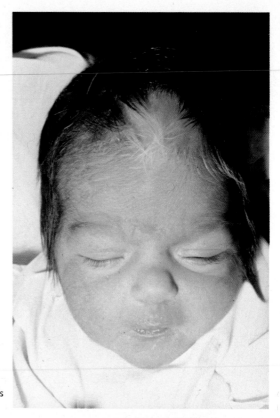

94. White forelock of Waardenburg's
syndrome

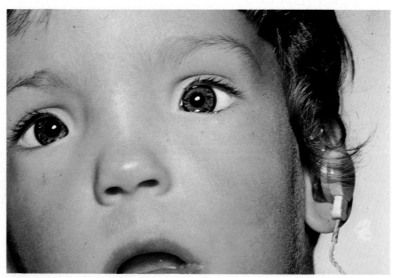

95. Heterochromia iris and dystopia
canthorum in Waardenburg's syndrome

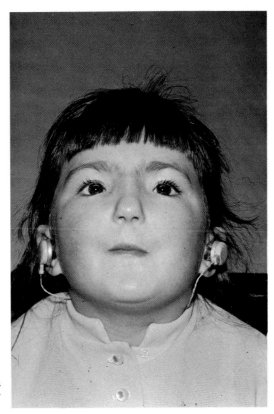

96. Confluent eyebrows, dystopia canthorum and deafness of Waardenburg's syndrome

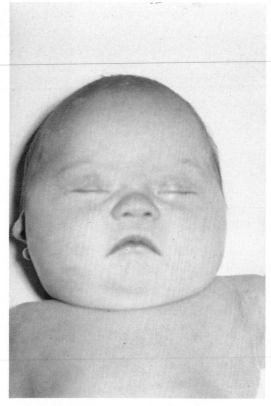

97. Down's trisomy-21

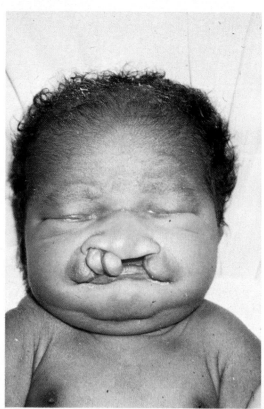

98. Patau's trisomy-13

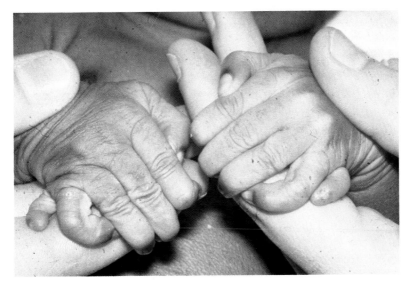

99. Polydactyly in trisomy-13

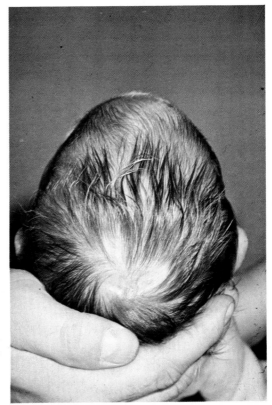

100. Partial thickness scalp defect in trisomy-13

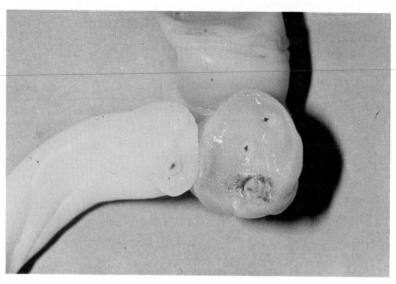

101. Single umbilical artery in trisomy-13

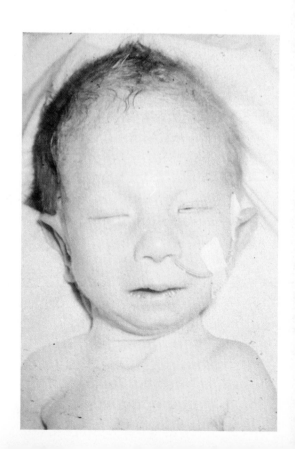

102. Edwards's trisomy-18

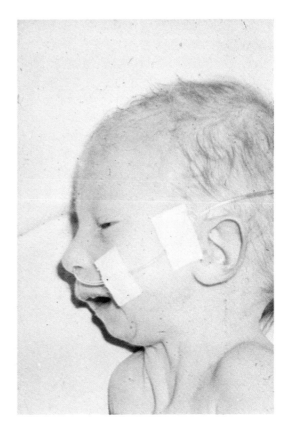

103. Edwards's trisomy-18

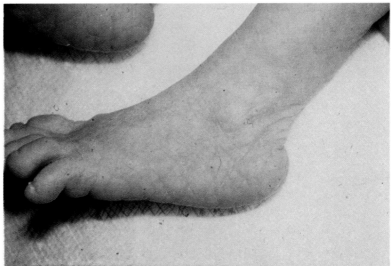

104. 'Rocker bottom' feet in Edwards's
trisomy-18

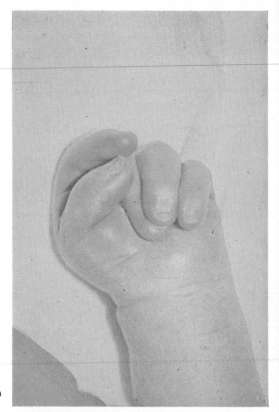

105. Overlapping finger posture in Edwards's trisomy-18

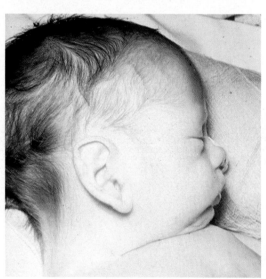

106. Neck webbing in Turner's syndrome

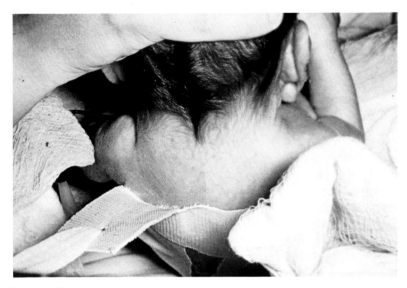

107. Low 'trident' hairline in Turner's
syndrome

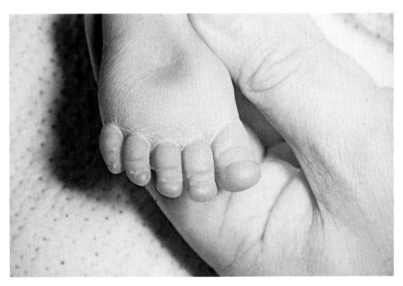

108. Congenital lymphoedema and
hypoplastic toenails in Turner's syndrome

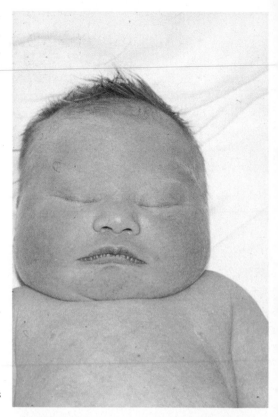

109. Congenital heart disease in Down's syndrome

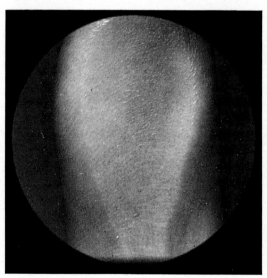

110. Low arch fingerprint pattern in Edwards's syndrome

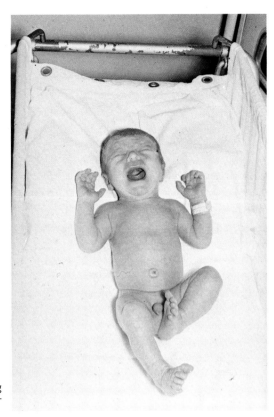

111. Growing dusky on vigorous crying suggests abnormality of the cardio-vascular system

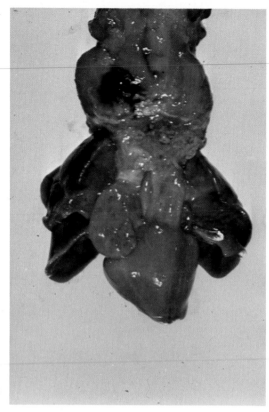

112. Lung hypoplasia in Potter's syndrome

The agencies involved are the doctors and their special ancillaries, the nurses, and the family.

113-115   The doctors

The initial situation is usually acute: the child needs an emergency operation by an expert; this is always serious in a small baby. In less urgent cases the special surgeon may come to the nursery to explain his policy for initial operation in cases such as cleft lip or palate. He reassures the mother that he has seen worse cases and can reinforce this with pictorial evidence of a good result (113, 114, 115). Interim visits will be made to his clinic and there she will meet the orthodontist and speech therapist on the team.

116-118

An operation may not be necessary, but the family still makes an early visit to an outside special centre, for instance to be told the schedule of limb prosthesis (116-118).

119-123

After an interval, some special investigations are carried out to detect possible covert associated congenital abnormalities (119: ureteric reflux and dilatation – the baby had an imperforate anus). Anticipatory surveillance is necessary where some aspects of multiple defect cannot be detected in the nursery (120: deafness in rubella embryopathy) and the early detection of such handicaps is important (121: deafness in cousins with Waardenburg's syndrome; the girl was diagnosed earlier and accepts the aid more readily). Some other defects do not begin to develop until months or years have passed (122: aniridia; the child will develop glaucoma, probably with cataract, and disorders such as Wilms' tumour or mental retardation with cerebellar ataxia may develop; 123: capillary naevus – may prove to be Sturge-Weber disease). Happily some things resolve spontaneously: testicles not uncommonly descend and a patent ductus or ventricular septal defect may close.

All children with abnormalities are notified to the Medical Officer of Health. They will be ascertained as having a definite handicap or being 'at risk' of developing one. Their likely needs are assessed and catered for, their educational needs in particular. Ideally, they will all maintain contact with the paediatric service and local authority and reports will be exchanged at intervals between these services and the family doctor.

124   Finally, it should be said that the ascertainment of
                                        certain abnormalities could only be counter-productive,
                                        for the reason that any possible trouble is very remote.
                                        Complete heart block (124) is an example; the only
                                        plan here is to tell the parents to inform any doctors
                                        who attend the child in later life about the condition.
                                        There is no need to adumbrate that it may or may
                                        not be a sleeper for some Stokes or Adams of the
                                        21st century.

11, 125, 126 The nurses   Special skills enter into diagnosis as well as management,
                                        and especially affect the quality of the survivor. The
                                        good nurse recognises imperforate anus in the delivery
                                        room and a urine bag is instantly applied (125);
                                        meconium in the urine points to fistula. Excessive
                                        bubbly mucus on delivery (11), especially after
                                        hydramnios, is the first danger sign of oesophageal
                                        atresia; the nursing plan, which covers several hours,
                                        is to suck the baby out and continue doing so until
                                        he is delivered to the special cardiothoracic unit. Here
                                        the local nurse continues suction until the baby arrives
                                        in the theatre. In cases of cleft palate the plan may
                                        cover several days. The early (spoon) feeding can be
                                        so messy that it may be better to let the experienced
                                        nurse cope with it. The mother can attend and need
                                        not feel inadequate if she knows that she will take over
                                        in a couple of days when the baby is 'broken in'. The
                                        plan may sometimes cover weeks or months. With
                                        Pierre Robin syndrome for instance, the child must be
                                        saved from suffocation (126) and has to stay in hospital
                                        until he can safely lie in the supine position.

127   The parents   The parents' function is to continue or to supplement
                                        the measures instituted by the nurses or ancillary
                                        specialists. It may simply be the use of a special bottle-
                                        teat in a case of cleft palate prior to surgery (127), the
                                        management of surgical stomata, or ensuring the
                                        patency of hydrocephalus valves. There is an encouraging
                                        trend to early enlistment of the parents for instruction
                                        in the planned management of conditions such as tonic
                                        and postural disorders or blindness.

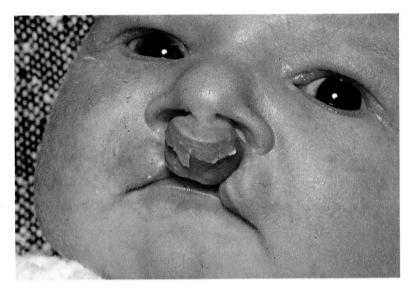

113. Cleft lip before repair

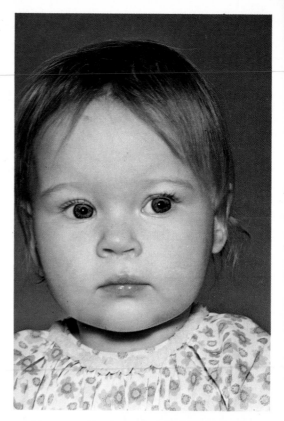

114.   Cleft lip after surgical repair

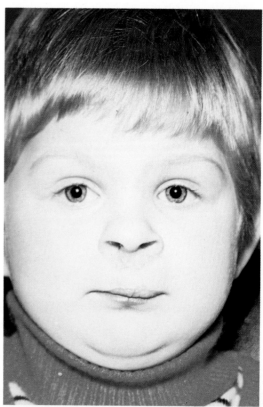

115.   Cleft lip after surgical repair

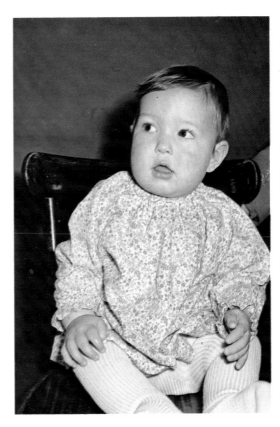

116. Limb prosthesis

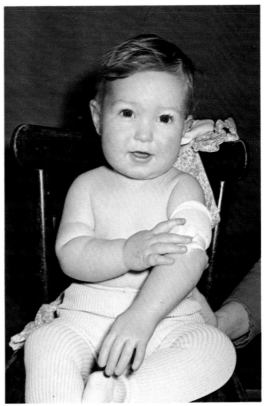

117. Limb prosthesis

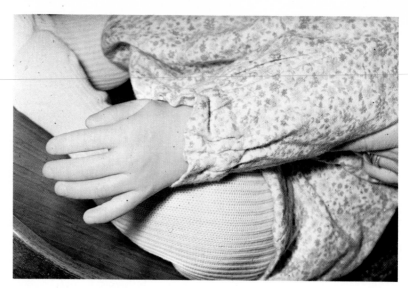

118. Limb prosthesis

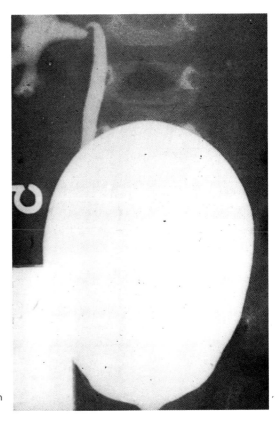

119. Ureteric reflux associated with imperforate anus

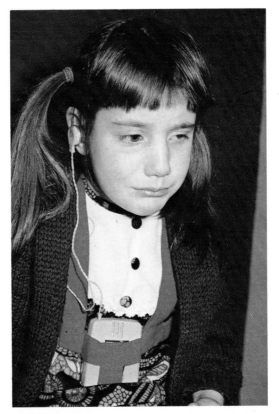

120. Deafness in rubella embryopathy

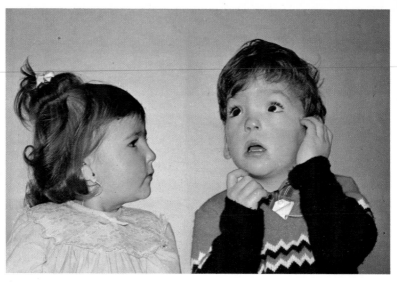

121. Deafness   in   cousins   with
Waardenburg's syndrome

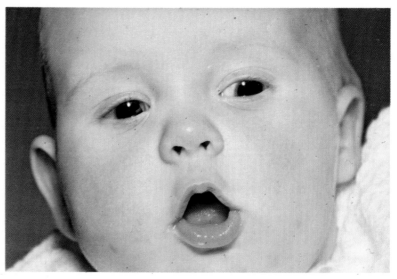

122. Aniridia

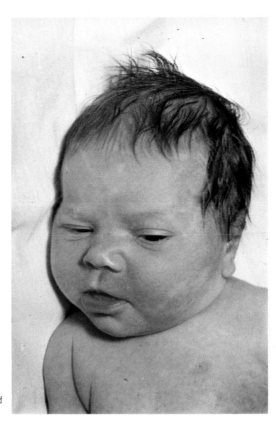

123. Capillary naevus possibly associated with Sturge-Weber disease

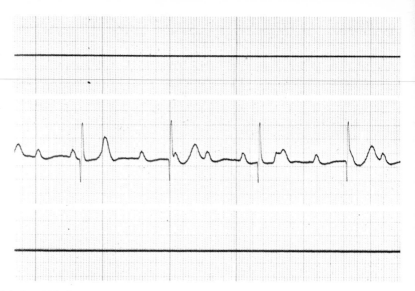

124. Complete heart block

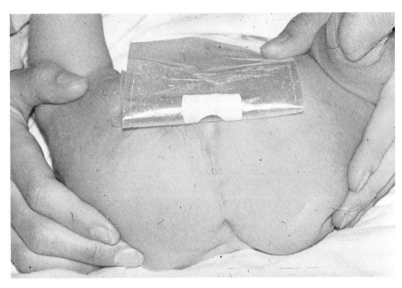

125. Urine bag instantly applied when imperforate anus is recognised

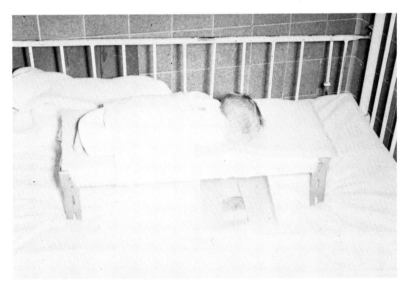

126. Prevention of suffocation in Pierre Robin syndrome

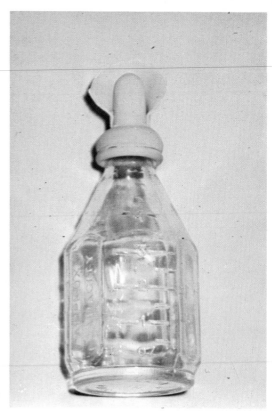

127. Special bottle teat for use with
cleft palate prior to surgery

121, 128-131

Families readily appreciate the genetic determination of defects already present in one parent or some close relative (128, 129: father and son; 130, 131: siblings with microcephaly; 121: Waardenburg's syndrome in cousins). Sometimes causal relationships may be defined, as with rubella, intrauterine compression or drug therapy.

Usually the doctor explains a genetic mutation as 'just one of those things'. However, he should always ask the parents why *they* thought the abnormality occurred. They often need to be disabused of some misconception; for instance they have to be assured that cleft palate is not caused by accidental haemorrhage or that achondroplasia is not the outcome of consanguinity. The discussion should finally touch on whether the abnormality could have been prevented.

Could it happen again?

All parents wonder about this and the question must always be discussed with them. Very many forms of congenital abnormality are liable to recur and the risks can be precisely estimated. On most cases encountered in the nursery the informed clinician is a competent adviser. Nevertheless, misinformation is still rife: the uninformed doctor tends to be over-optimistic and the lay person over-pessimistic.

130-133

The arithmetically elementary genetic advice is generally grave, as when straightforward recessive (130, 131: microcephaly in siblings) or dominant (132: achondroplastic mother with achondroplastic baby) genes operate. Advice is also easy to give on conditions like Down's syndrome or spina bifida, although they are more complex genetically; the facts have become familiar to the paediatricians because of their high frequency in the population. Reference to a simple manual of genetic advice will tell the clinician whether he can easily explain the less common conditions, or needs the help of a genetic consultant.

Finally, however clearly the highest risk is conveyed the most intrepid parents will not be deterred (133).

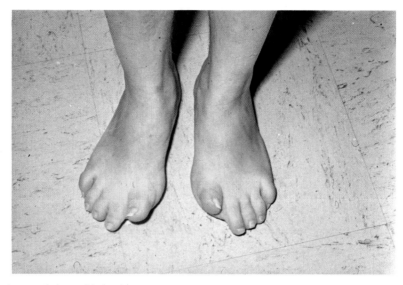

128. Webbed toes, father of baby in
plate 129

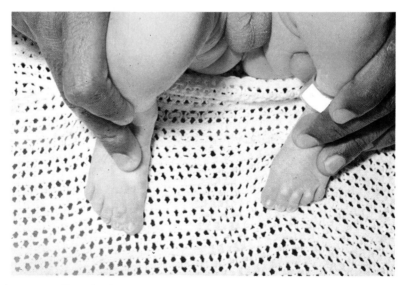

129. Webbed toes, son of man in plate 128

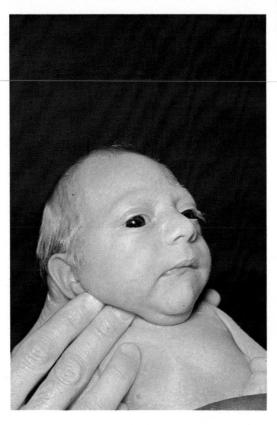

130. Microcephaly, sibling of baby in plate 131

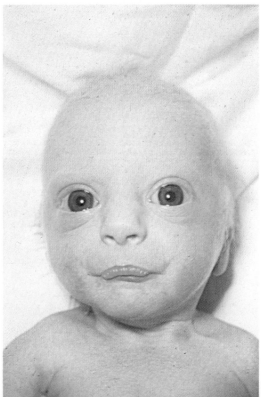

131. Microcephaly, sibling of baby in plate 130

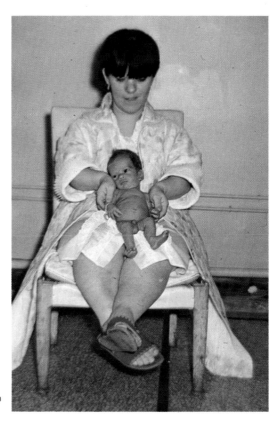

132. Achondroplastic mother with achondroplastic baby

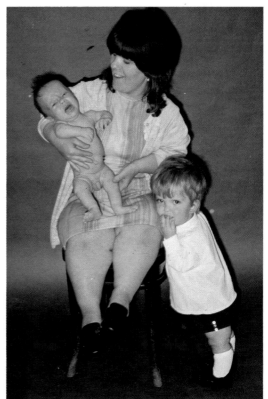

133. The same achondroplastic mother as in plate 132, with a second achondroplastic baby

Section six

Skin defects

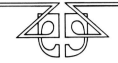

Minor abnormalities of the skin have been discussed in several of the earlier volumes of this Atlas. They occur most commonly among trivial complaints in the routine care of babies who are well, about 3 per cent of whom are affected by vascular and pigmented naevi. Their most important occurrence, however, is in connection with congenital abnormality.

In discussing even the most innocuous of blemishes, it is inexcusable to try to fob off the mother with the non-explanation that 'it is nothing'. It has rightly been said that this is the doctor talking to himself; he should instead describe the lesion in simple terms and give a proper explanation along these lines; 'this is not serious, there is no risk to the baby, so we need do no special tests nor give any treatment; in due course it will either go away completely or be inconspicuous. Even if it does leave some mark we can then do something simple to disperse it or conceal it if you like.'

1-3

A trivial abnormality in the skin may be the indicator or harbinger of serious abnormality elsewhere. For example, a pigmented hairy naevus (1) was found to be associated with an umbilical varix (2), and on the following day the baby developed heart-failure (3) due to transposition of the great vessels.

4

Apparently isolated trivial defects must be accorded proper respect in 'danger zones' such as the line of neural tube closure (4: two siblings had severe spina bifida; minor lesions at this site demand close attention).

The types of defect recognised in the nursery are:

1. Vascular birthmarks
2. Pigmented birthmarks
3. Partial thickness defects
4. Keratinisation disorders
5. Blistering and bullous disorders
6. Neuroectodermal dysplasias

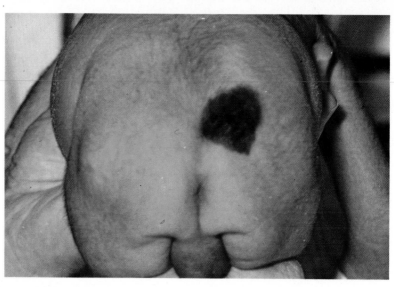

1. This pigmented hairy naevus was
an indicator of serious abnormality
elsewhere

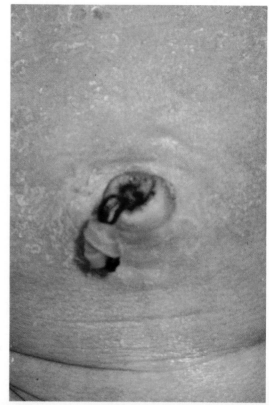

2. Umbilical varix in the same baby
as in plate 1

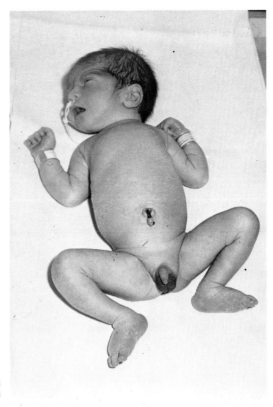

3. Heart failure due to transposition of the great vessels in the same baby as in plate 1

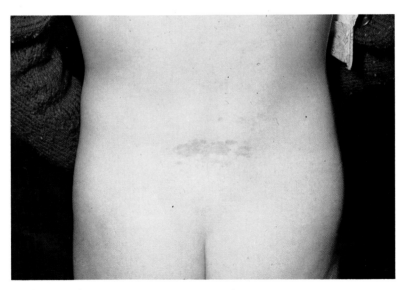

4. Minor lesion in the lumbar region; two siblings had severe spina bifida

| 5-11 | Capillary haemangiomas | Capillary haemangiomas are flat or slightly raised lesions caused by dilated capillaries in the superficial layers of the dermis. About 50 per cent of babies have physiological 'stork marks' and the denser *naevus flammeus* is also common on the face and head (5, 6, 7). It blanches easily on pressure (8) and the blood rushes back quickly. Lesions on the trunk and limbs may be extensive (9, 10, 11). |

| 12-31 | Cavernous haemangiomas | Cavernous haemangiomas are conspicuous raised lesions which often do not appear until the baby is a few weeks old; they may be multiple (12) and sometimes seem to cluster (13). Their location in the skin may be quite superficial (14, 15, 16) or they may be more or less deeply buried (17, 18, 19, 20, 21, 22). The term 'strawberry naevus' is most applicable when there are hair follicles on the swelling (23). The vast majority can be dealt with conservatively. The main problem is to convince the parents and support them if the larger haemangiomas are traumatised with consequent ulceration, haemorrhage and infection (24, 25, 26, 27). The ultimate outlook is good; islands of epithelium will form and spread to coalesce and cover the area with whole skin, and finally the swelling will subside and disappear (28, 29, 30, 31). |

| 32-35 | | Deeper structures may be involved in either type of haemangiomatous malformation and some rare clinical conditions have been defined, e.g. Klippel-Trenaunay syndrome with capillary haemangioma (32, 33) and Maffucci's syndrome with cavernous haemangioma. Cystic hygroma (34) is a lymphangiomatous swelling with the unique characteristic of brilliant transillumination (35). |

| 36-41 | Hereditary telangiectasia, Osler-Rendu-Weber disease | Hereditary telangiectasia, Osler-Rendu-Weber disease, can present in infancy not with telangiectases but with cavernous haemangiomas (36, 37); this baby was diagnosed in the nursery because of rectal bleeding (38); the new lesions cropping at four months (39, 40) and at two years were still exclusively haemangiomas (41). |

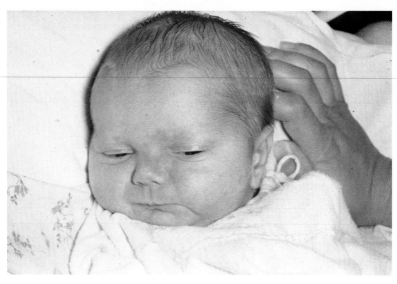

5. Capillary naevus on the face

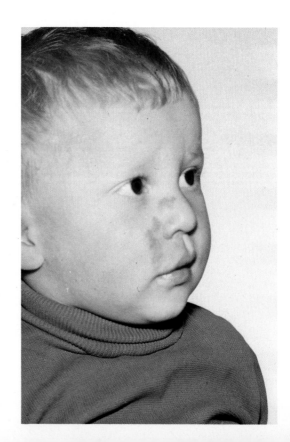

6. Capillary naevus on the face

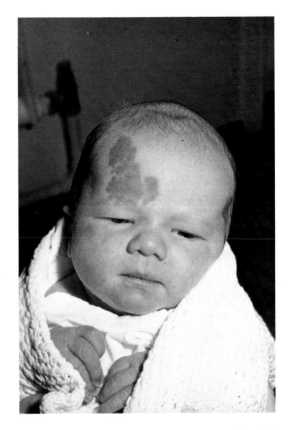

7. Capillary naevus on the face

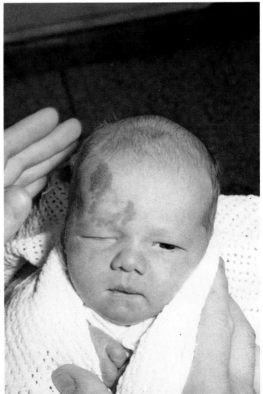

8. Blanching on pressure of capillary naevus

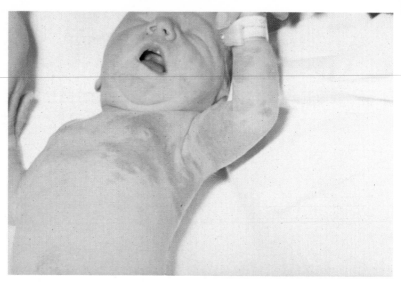

9. Capillary naevus of the trunk and
arm

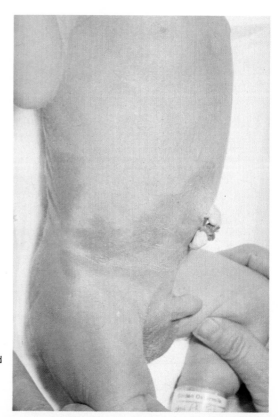

10. Capillary naevus of the trunk and
leg

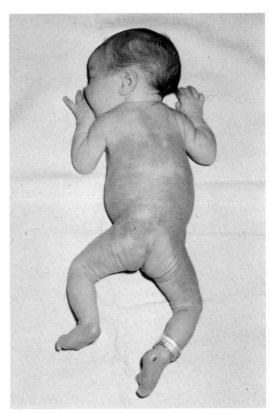

11. Capillary naevus of the trunk and legs

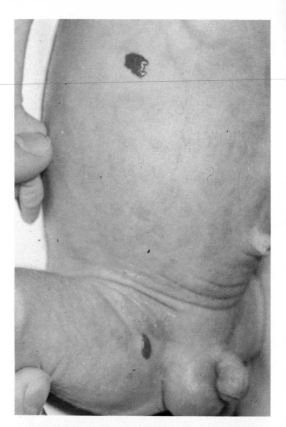

12. Multiple cavernous haemangiomas

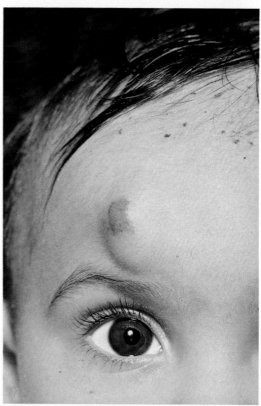

13. Clustered cavernous haemangiomas

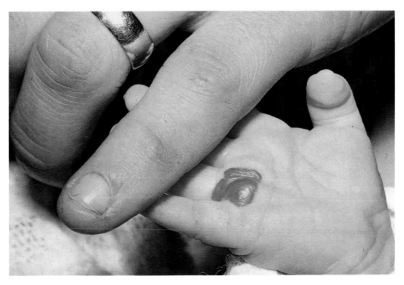

14. Superficial cavernous haemangioma

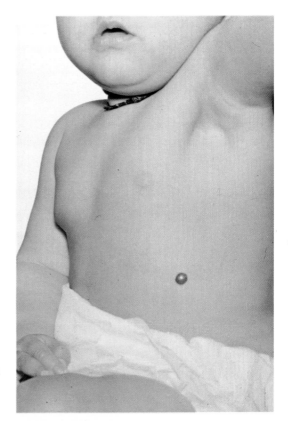

15. Superficial cavernous haemangioma

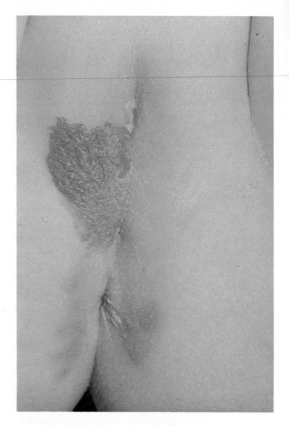

16. Superficial cavernous haemangioma

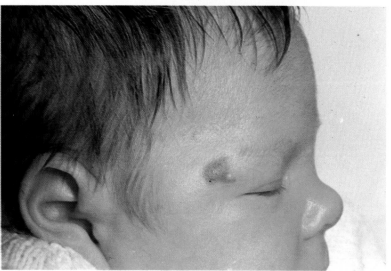

17. Deeply buried cavernous haemangioma

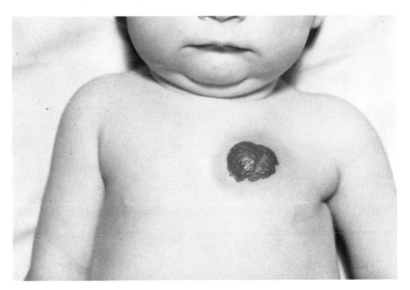

18. Deeply buried cavernous haemangioma

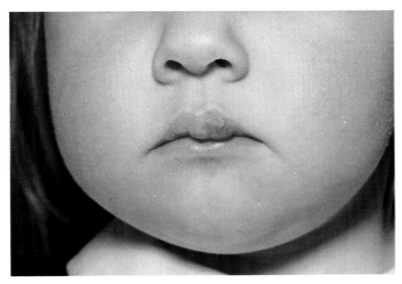

19. Deeply buried cavernous haemangioma

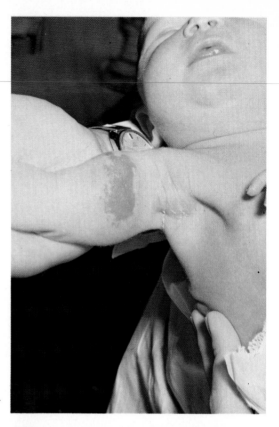

20. Deeply buried cavernous haemangioma

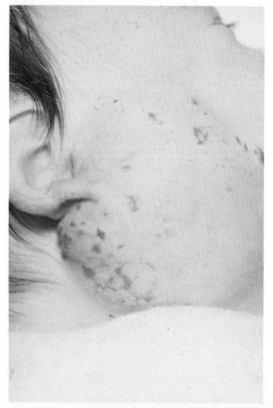

21. Deeply buried cavernous haemangioma

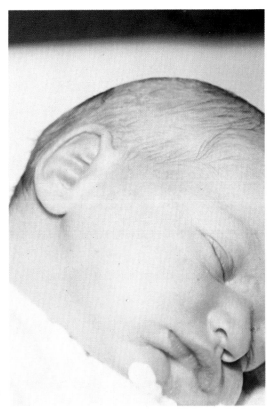

22. Deeply buried cavernous haemangioma

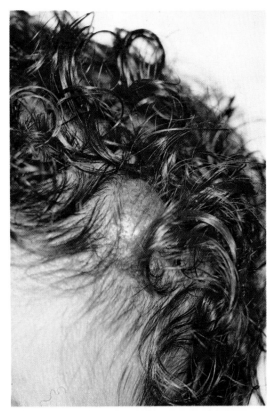

23. Strawberry naevus

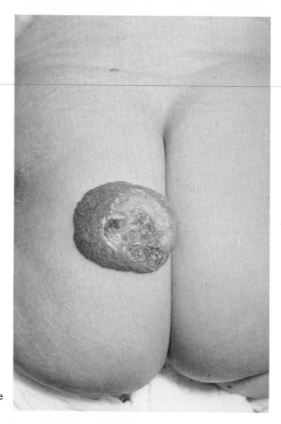

24. Ulceration and infection of a large
haemangioma

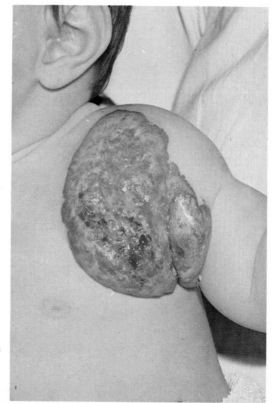

25. Ulceration and infection of a large
haemangioma

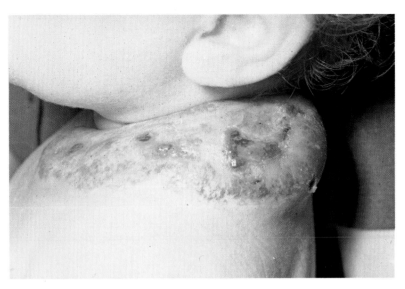

26. Ulceration and infection of a large haemangioma

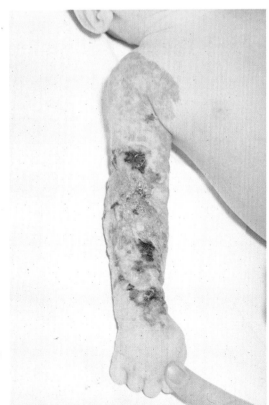

27. Ulceration and infection of a large haemangioma

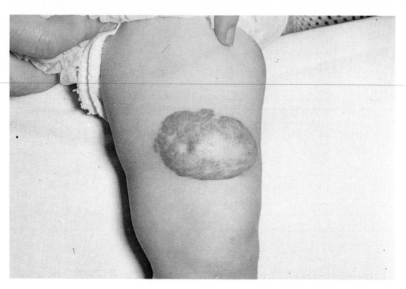

28. Epithelium coalescing to cover the haemangioma

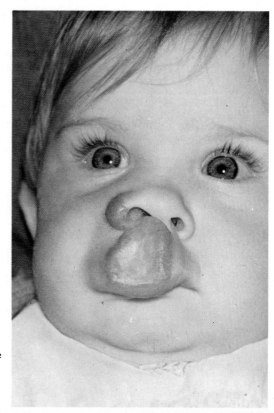

29. Haemangioma covered with whole skin

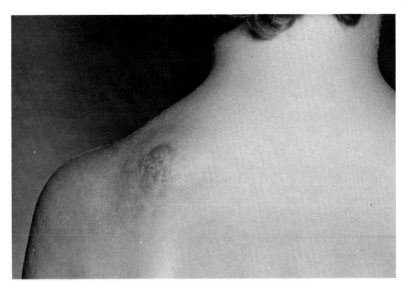

30. Swelling of a haemangioma almost
completely subsided

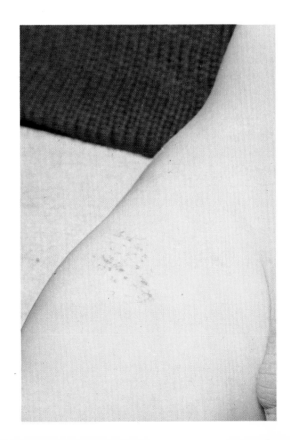

31. Haemangioma almost invisible

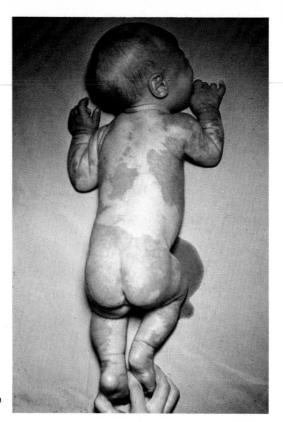

32. Klippel-Trenaunay syndrome with
capillary haemangioma

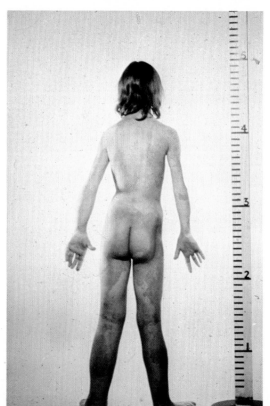

33. Klippel-Trenaunay syndrome with
capillary haemangioma

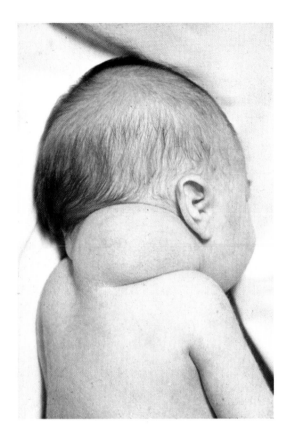

34. Cystic hygroma

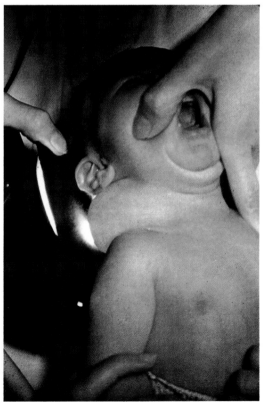

35. Transillumination of cystic hygroma

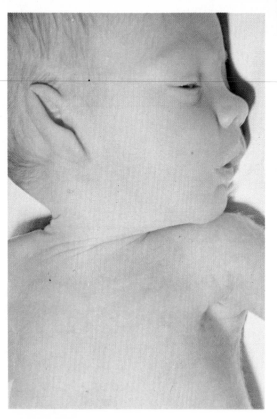

36. Osler-Rendu-Weber disease

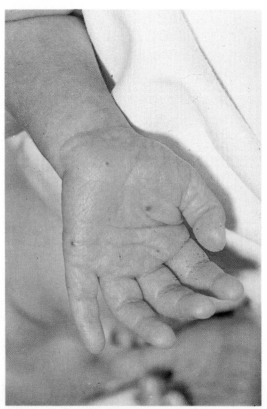

37. Osler-Rendu-Weber disease

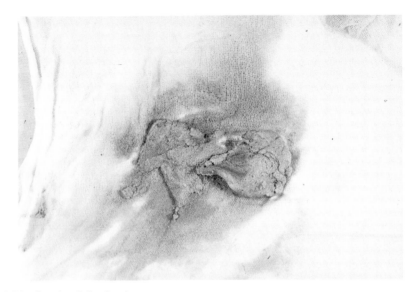

38. Rectal bleeding in Osler-Rendu-Weber disease

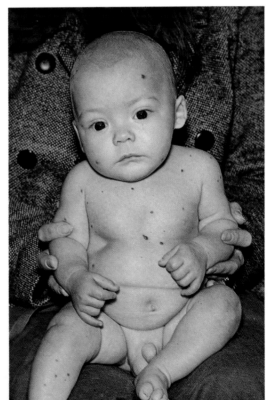

39. New haemangiomas appearing at four months in Osler-Rendu-Weber disease

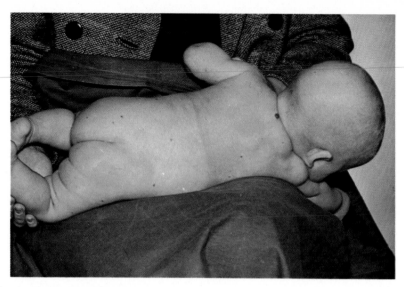

40. New haemangiomas appearing at
four months in Osler-Rendu-Weber
disease

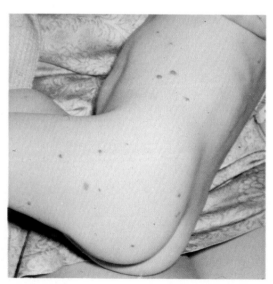

41. New haemangiomas appearing at
two years in Osler-Rendu-Weber disease

1, 42-54

These show a wide range in depth of colour (42-50) and are usually, though not always, homogeneous (51). If the lesion is palpable, it is called either *naevus molle* or cellular naevus (52). A few are hairy at birth (1) while others grow hairy later on (53, 54).

55-57

Malignant melanoma can be congenital and the darker naevi may need biopsy if they are growing rapidly or if there is any indication of extension. This is particularly so if they are multiple (55, 56, 57: these were benign 'juvenile melanomas').

The dominant mode of inheritance of von Recklinghausen's neurofibromatosis has led to the observation that the presence of more than half a dozen pigmented naevi at birth may be the earliest indication of the disorder.

58-61

The pigmented naevi of infantile urticaria pigmentosa are usually inconspicuous in the nursery and not recognised for a few months (58). They contain mast cells which release histamine on pressure, causing a wheal (59, 60). Dermatographia may develop (61).

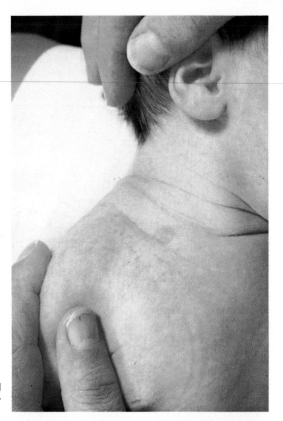

42. Single, light coloured, pigmented birthmark; the mother had neuro-fibromatosis

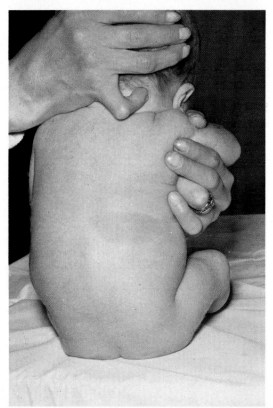

43. Light coloured pigmented birth-mark

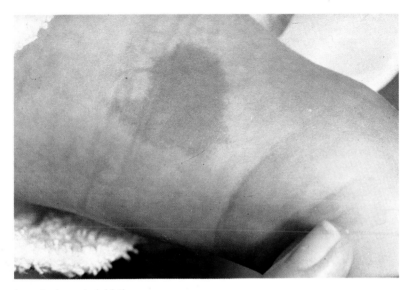

44. Light coloured pigmented birthmark

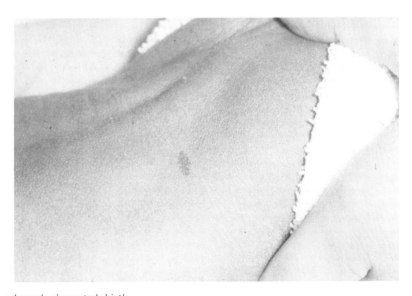

45. Light coloured pigmented birthmark

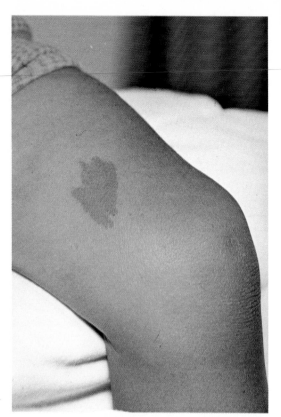

46. Medium coloured pigmented birthmark

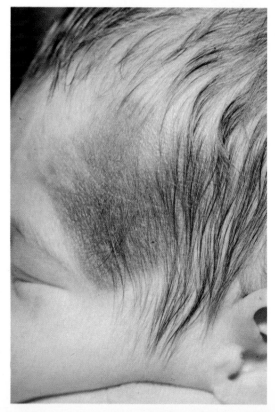

47. Medium coloured pigmented birthmark

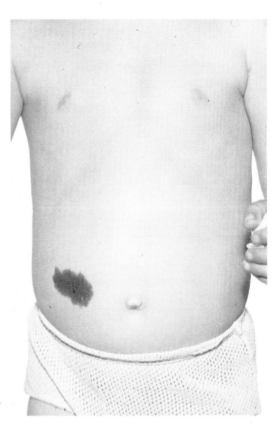

48. Dark coloured pigmented birthmark

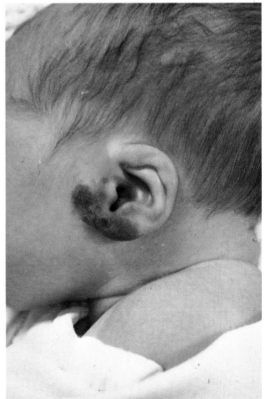

49. Dark coloured pigmented birthmark

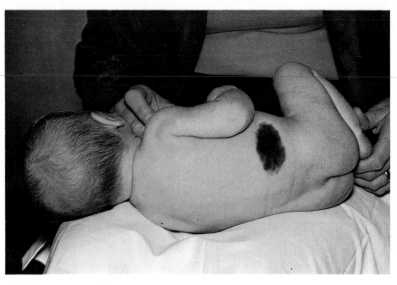

50. Dark coloured pigmented birthmark

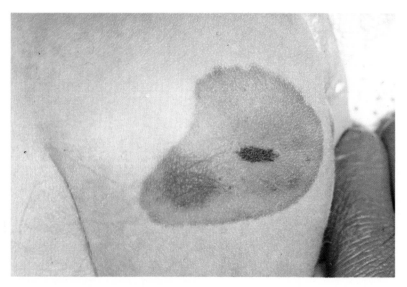

51. Heterogeneous depth of colour in
a pigmented birthmark

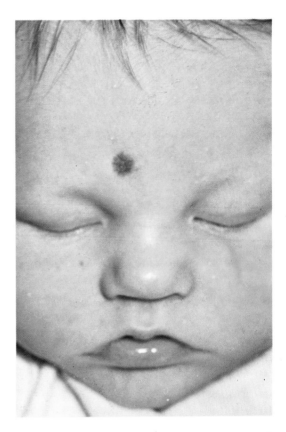

52. *Naevus molle*

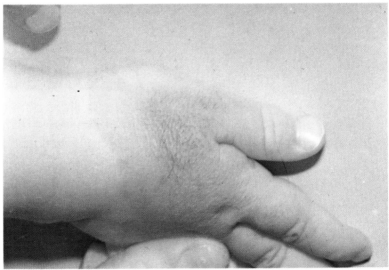

53. Light coloured birthmark which grew hairy after birth

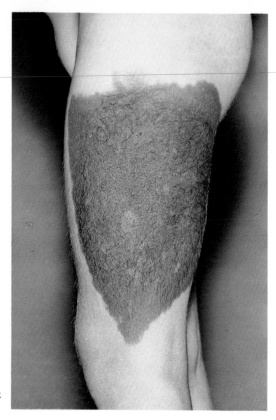

54. Large, dark pigmented birthmark
which grew hairy after birth

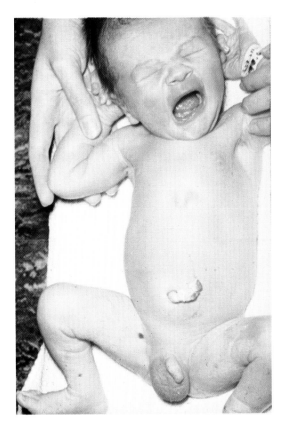

55. Benign juvenile melanoma

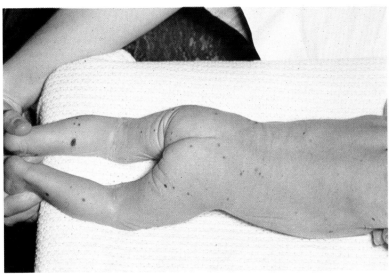

56. Benign juvenile melanoma

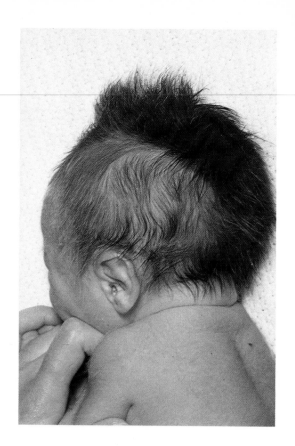

57. Benign juvenile melanoma

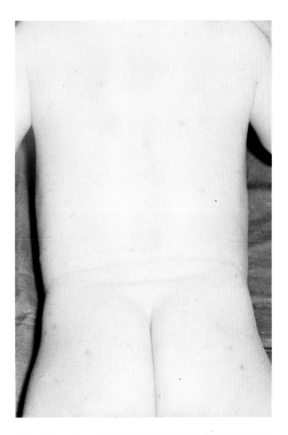

58. Infantile urticaria pigmentosa

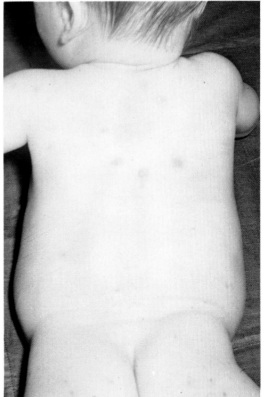

59. Wheals on pressure in infantile
urticaria pigmentosa

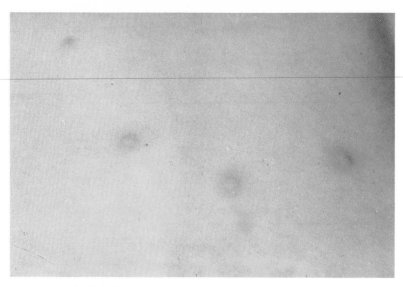

60. Wheals on pressure in infantile
urticaria pigmentosa

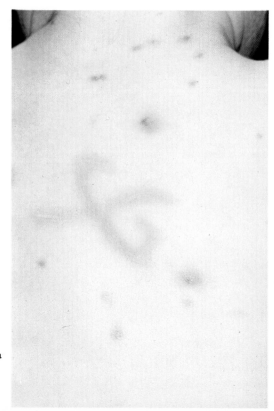

61. Dermatographia   in   urticaria
pigmentosa

Partial thickness defects

62-73

These are usually superficial (62, 63) but if they go deep the underlying structures are sometimes visible through a fine membrane. If there is a granulating or exudative surface it forms crusts which must be softened and removed, and the end result is inconspicuous (64, 65, 66, 67, 68, 69, 70, 71). A favourite site is the scalp, where they can cause a bald spot (72, 73).

74, 75

Sometimes amniotic adhesion to the edge of these defects occurs. This is now thought to be secondary rather than causative, and the relationship with 'congenital gangrene' (74) and cicatrisation (75) is a matter for speculation.

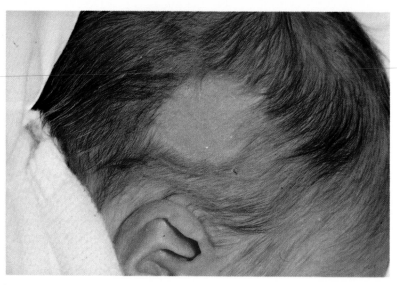

62. Superficial partial thickness skin
defect of the scalp

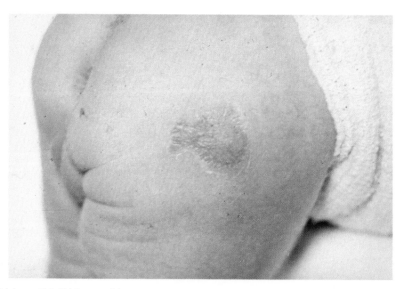

63. Superficial partial thickness skin
defect of the buttock

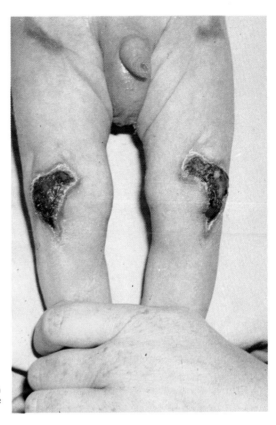

64. Deeper partial thickness skin defect of the knees with exudative surface

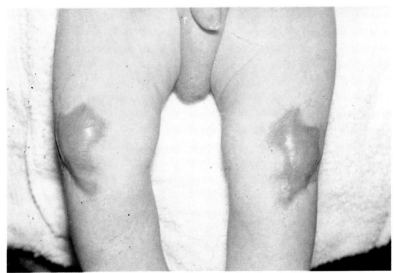

65. Knees of the infant in plate 64 partially healed

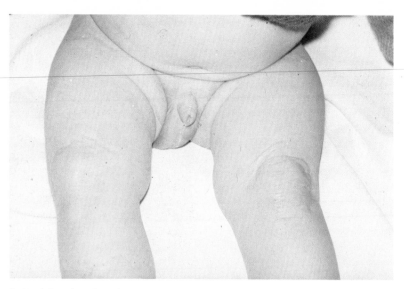

66. Knees of the infant in plate 64 completely healed

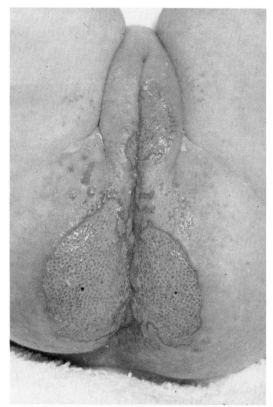

67. Partial thickness skin defect of the perianal region with granulatory surface

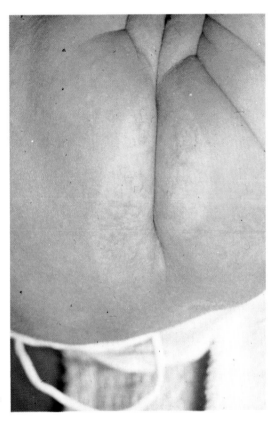

68. Epithelium coalescing over the defective area shown in plate 67

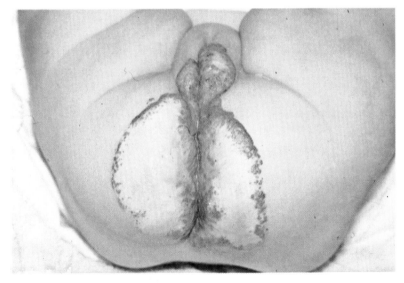

69. Vascularisation around the defective area shown in plate 67

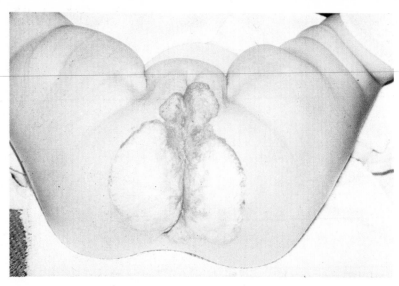

70. Fading of the mark in the perianal
area shown in plate 67

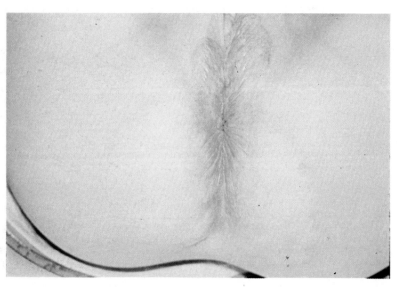

71. Result of complete healing of the
perianal area shown in plate 67

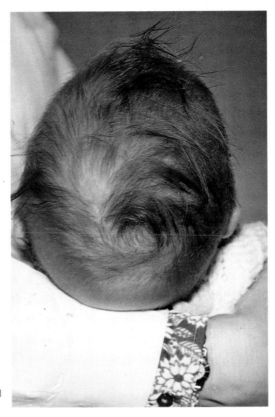

72. Bald spot resulting from a partial thickness skin defect of the scalp

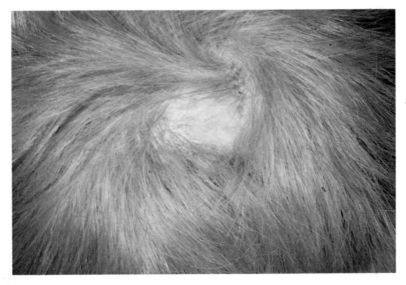

73. Bald patch resulting from a partial thickness skin defect of the scalp

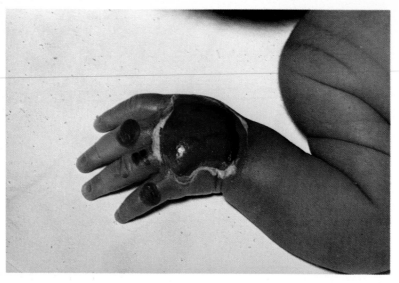

74. Congenital gangrene

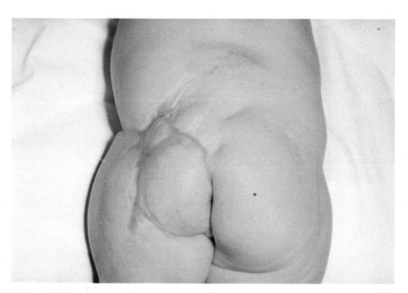

75. Congenital cicatrisation

Ichthyotic changes at birth are most likely to be seen in *ichthyosis congenita* – 'collodion skin' (76, 77). There is a shiny yellow-brown investing membrane which splits off in sheets over a few days (78, 79). This process may reveal a normal integument (80). Some babies with this condition, however, develop non-bullous ichthyosiform erythroderma, although this more commonly occurs without any preceding 'collodion skin'.

The much rarer *ichthyosis fetalis* results in the 'harlequin fetus', a grotesque disorder incompatible with survival and in no way related to the physiological harlequin colour change.

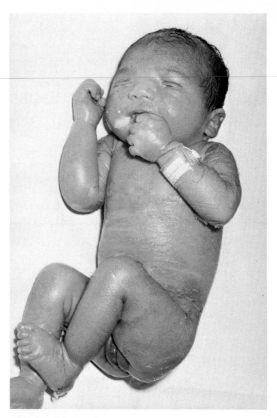

76. *Ichthyosis congenita*

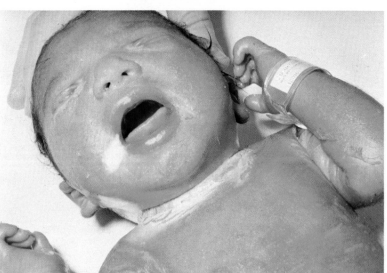

77. *Ichthyosis congenita*

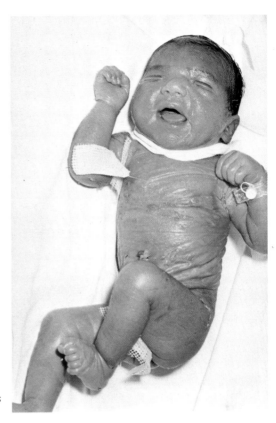

78. Collodion membrane of *ichthyosis congenita*

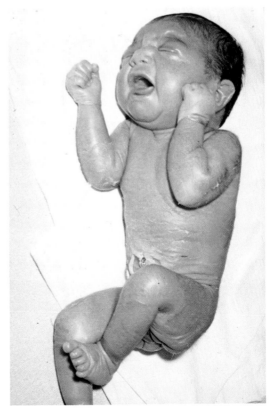

79. Collodion membrane of *ichthyosis congenita*

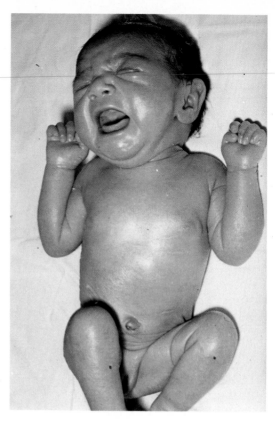

80. Normal skin revealed after loss of the collodion membrane of *ichthyosis congenita*

81-86

Blisters present at birth are most probably caused by epidermolysis bullosa (81) or the bullous form of congenital ichthyosiform erythroderma. In the latter, the blisters appear on areas of erythroderma (82), but careful inspection discovers some areas of ichthyosis (83). The blisters heal rapidly, and this process is accelerated by steroids (84: 5 weeks). After weeks or months a generalised hyperkeratosis is established; its elements are more friable and greasy than in the nonbullous form of the disorder (85: 6 months; 86: 6 years).

Incontinentia pigmenti is considered with the neuroectodermal dysplasias.

The bullous form of keratosis follicularis (Darier's disease) is the only other likely cause of congenital blisters but it is exceptionally rare.

87-89

It is important to differentiate Ritter's toxic epidermal necrolysis. This is not congenital but of late onset (87: 2 weeks); the illness is due to the baby's toxic response to phage-specific staphylococcal infection and the skin rubs off in sheets (88, 89). In successfully treated cases the skin is clear by the end of the neonatal period.

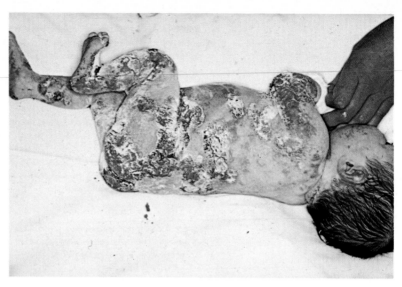

81. Epidermolysis bullosa

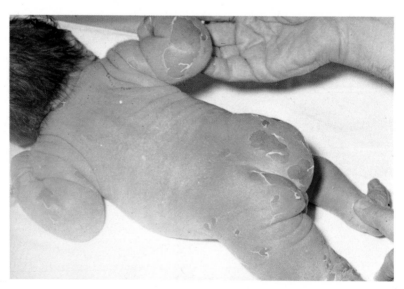

82. Bullous form of congenital ichthyosiform erythoderma

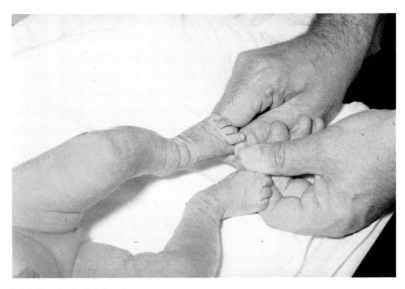

83. Areas of ichthyosis in ichthyosiform erythoderma

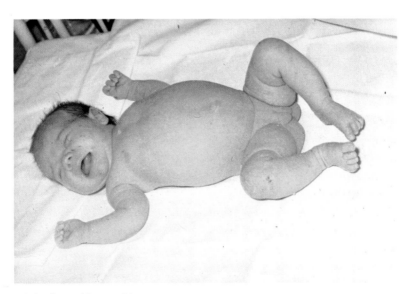

84. Accelerated healing with steroid
therapy; at 5 weeks

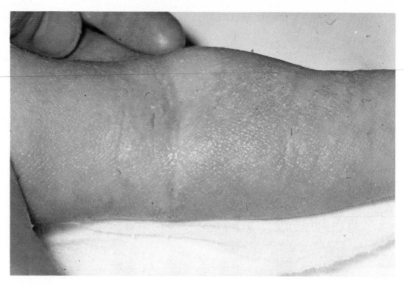

85. Subsequent generalised hyperkeratosis at 6 months

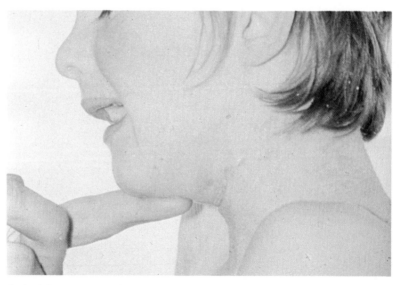

86. Hyperkeratosis at 6 years

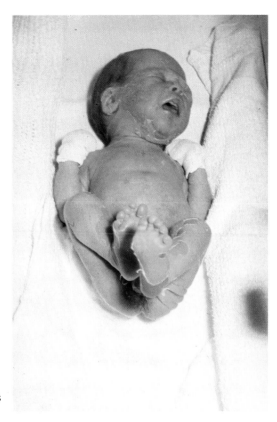

87. Ritter's toxic epidermal necrolysis at 2 weeks

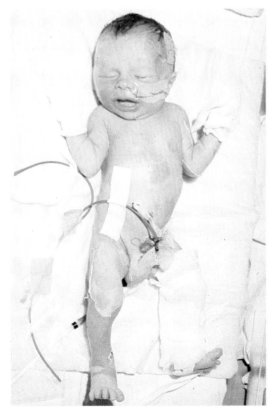

88. Ritter's toxic epidermal necrolysis

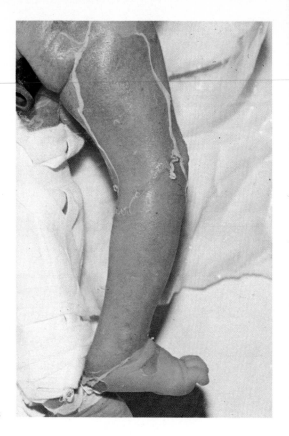

89. Ritter's toxic epidermal necrolysis

90-98

Sturge-Weber disease, which is the most common, can occur in the baby with a capillary naevus involving the territory of the first or second division of the trigeminal nerve (90). The likelihood of this is greater when similar naevi occur on the trunk and limbs (91, 92) especially if there is hypertrophy (93: right upper limb affected). The ipsilateral cerebral hemisphere has a vascular malformation (94) that restricts its growth (95: age 6 weeks, reduced volume of right hemicranium, thickened vault). Ultimately there is radio-opacity caused by a combination of calcification and ferrugination (96, 97; 'tramline' calcification). Buphthalmos (98: 3 months) is more likely when the ophthalmic division is affected; other eye lesions may be associated.

99-111

Incontinentia pigmenti (Bloch-Sulzberger) is usually classified among the blistering disorders present at birth (99, 100). There are, however, frequent congenital ocular lesions, and severe neonatal neurological deficit has been linked with cerebral malformation (101: polymicrogyria; 102: hypoplastic pyramidal tract). The blisters may cluster in bizarre arrangements if they are numerous (103, 104: 'Chinese lettering'), and afterwards they become crusted (105). The final pigmented stage has a splashed appearance (106). Fading occurs gradually (107: 6 months; 108: 1 year; 109, 110: 9 years) and is usually complete by the age of twenty. There may be, however, an ectodermal stigma in the form of dental anomaly (111: missing teeth, conical deformity). The condition is almost exclusive to the female, the vesicle fluid is eosinophil-laden, and there is often concomitant blood eosinophilia in the neonate.

42

Von Recklinghausen's neurofibromatosis may present multiple lightly-pigmented birthmarks. These are generally overlooked unless one parent has the disorder or a baby is very spotty (42: harmless single pigmented birthmark which was observed only after a careful search undertaken because the mother had neurofibromatosis).

112-114

Tuberose sclerosis does not develop the classical cutaneous disorder of epiloia (112) for several years but this may be preceded by the appearance of areas of depigmentation (113: achromic naevi; 114: characteristic leaf shape). It is not clear how often these are present at birth – a reflection of the current lack of knowledge about the natural history of congenital skin defects in general.

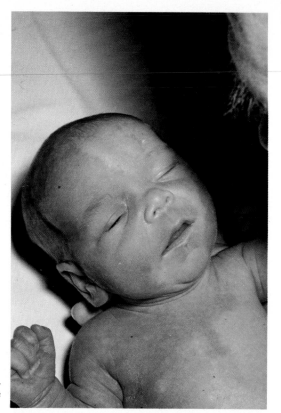

90. Sturge-Weber disease with capillary naevus of the territory of the trigeminal nerve

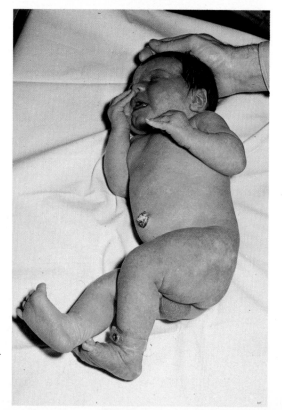

91. Sturge-Weber disease with capillary naevi on the face, trunk and limbs

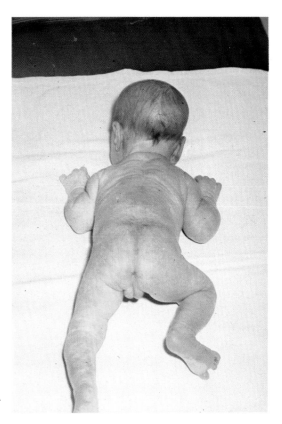

92. Sturge-Weber disease with capillary naevi on the face, trunk and limbs

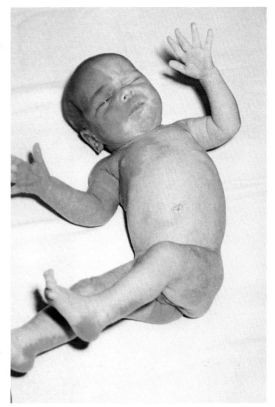

93. Sturge-Weber disease with hypertrophy of the right upper limb

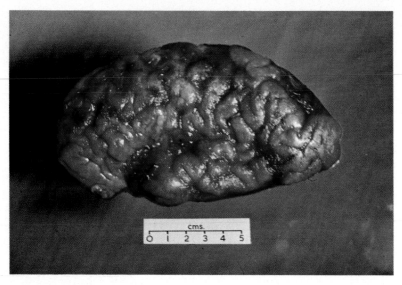

94. Cerebral vascular malformation in Sturge-Weber disease

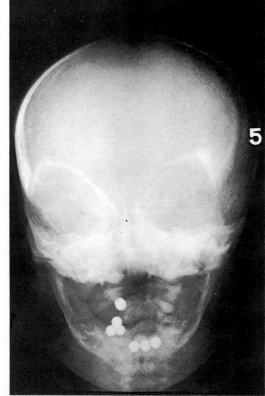

95. Sturge-Weber disease; roentgenogram of the skull at 6 weeks shows vault is smaller on right side with thickened inner table

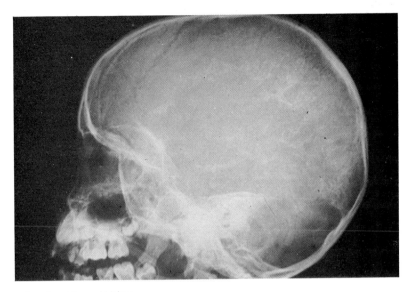

96. Radio-opacity in Sturge-Weber
disease

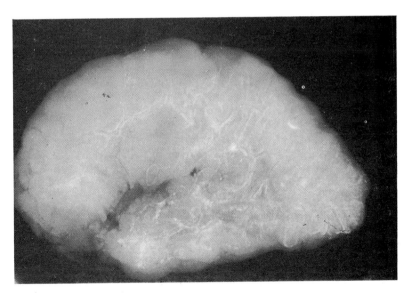

97. 'Tram-line' calcification in the
brain in Sturge-Weber disease

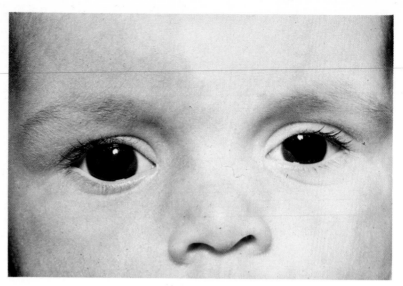

98. Buphthalmos at 3 months in
Sturge-Weber disease

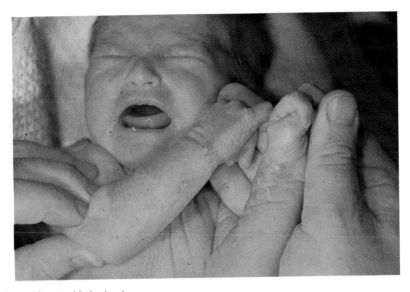

99. Blistering skin at birth in incontinentia pigmenti (Bloch-Sulzberger syndrome)

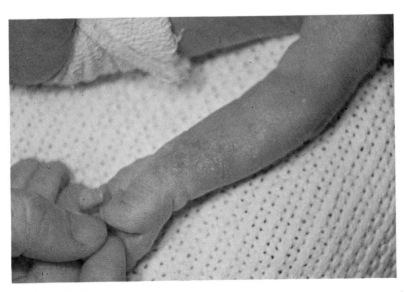

100. Blistering skin at birth in incontinentia pigmenti

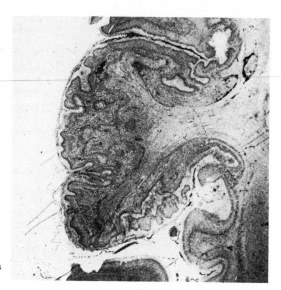

101. Polymicrogyria in incontinentia pigmenti

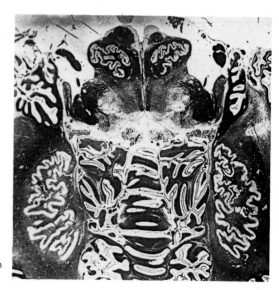

102. Hypoplastic pyramidal tract in incontinentia pigmenti

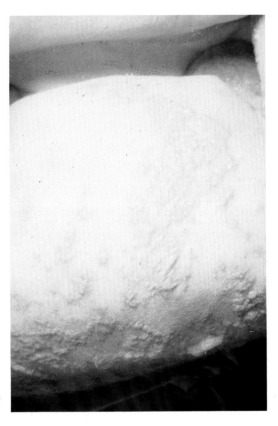

103. 'Chinese lettering' in incontinentia pigmenti

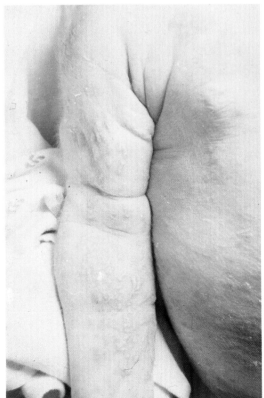

104. 'Chinese lettering' in incontinentia pigmenti

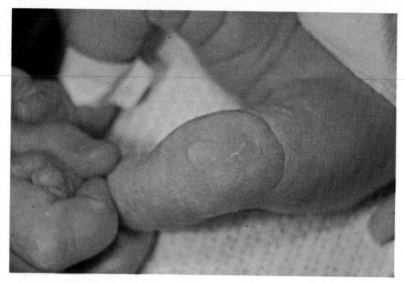

105. Crusting of lesions in incontinentia pigmenti

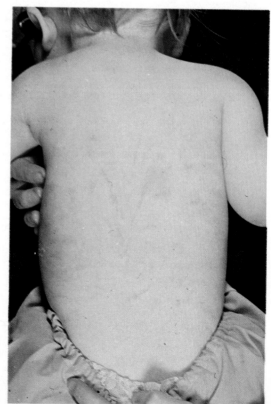

106. Splashed appearance of the final pigmented stage in incontinentia pigmenti

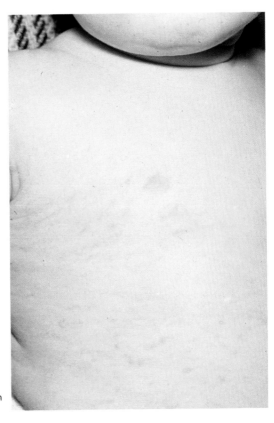

107. Gradual fading of the pigment in incontinentia pigmenti; 6 months

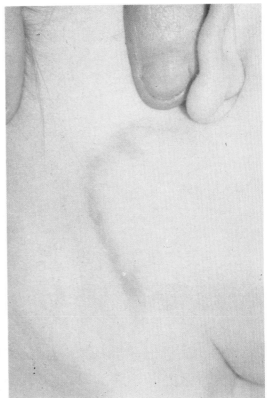

108. Gradual fading of the pigment in incontinentia pigmenti; 1 year

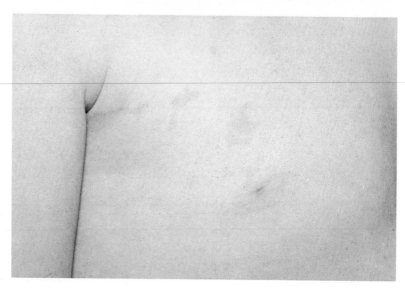

109. Fading of the pigment in incontinentia pigmenti; 9 years

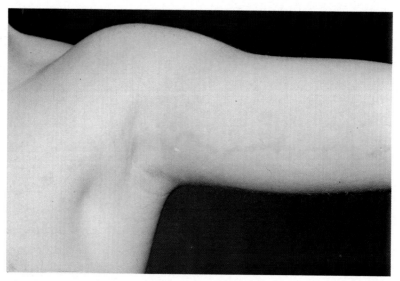

110. Fading of the pigment in incontinentia pigmenti; 9 years

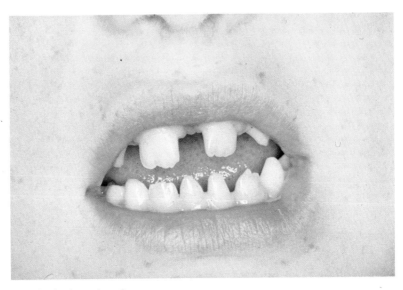

111. Dental anomaly in incontinentia pigmenti

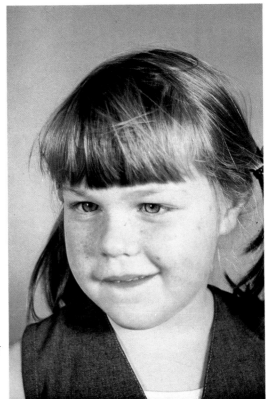

112. Classical cutaneous disorder of epiloia

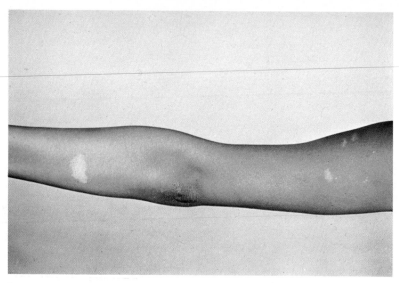

113. Achromic naevi in tuberose
sclerosis

114. Leaf-shaped achromic naevus in
tuberose sclerosis

Index

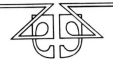

In this index page numbers are indicated in the normal way. The numbers shown in the brackets indicate the section in which an illustration will be found and its number within that section. Page numbers given alone refer to textual material.